T0235880

Health Informatics

This series is directed to healthcare professionals leading the transformation of healthcare by using information and knowledge. For over 20 years, Health Informatics has offered a broad range of titles: some address specific professions such as nursing, medicine, and health administration; others cover special areas of practice such as trauma and radiology; still other books in the series focus on interdisciplinary issues, such as the computer based patient record, electronic health records, and networked healthcare systems. Editors and authors, eminent experts in their fields, offer their accounts of innovations in health informatics. Increasingly, these accounts go beyond hardware and software to address the role of information in influencing the transformation of healthcare delivery systems around the world. The series also increasingly focuses on the users of the information and systems: the organizational, behavioral, and societal changes that accompany the diffusion of information technology in health services environments.

Developments in healthcare delivery are constant; in recent years, bioinformatics has emerged as a new field in health informatics to support emerging and ongoing developments in molecular biology. At the same time, further evolution of the field of health informatics is reflected in the introduction of concepts at the macro or health systems delivery level with major national initiatives related to electronic health records (EHR), data standards, and public health informatics.

These changes will continue to shape health services in the twenty-first century. By making full and creative use of the technology to tame data and to transform information, Health Informatics will foster the development and use of new knowledge in healthcare.

More information about this series at http://www.springer.com/series/1114

Ami B. Bhatt

Editor

Healthcare Information Technology for Cardiovascular Medicine

Telemedicine & Digital Health

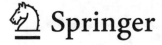 Springer

Editor
Ami B. Bhatt
Harvard Medical School, Massachusetts General Hospital
Boston, MA
USA

ISSN 1431-1917   ISSN 2197-3741   (electronic)
Health Informatics
ISBN 978-3-030-81032-0   ISBN 978-3-030-81030-6   (eBook)
https://doi.org/10.1007/978-3-030-81030-6

This Springer imprint is published by the registered company Springer Nature Switzerland AG
The registered company address is: Gewerbestrasse 11, 6330 Cham, Switzerland

Contents

Chapter 1
Telemedicine for Cardiovascular Disease Care

Ami B. Bhatt and Sandra Nagale

Telemedicine has become an essential mechanism for healthcare provision. We undertook this book prior to the COVID pandemic, which significantly changed the potential and future outlook for the implementation of virtual care worldwide.

Telemedicine is broadly defined as the "use of electronic information and telecommunications technologies to support and promote long-distance clinical health care, patient and professional health-related education, and public health and health administration" [5]. It is important to recognize that telehealth is not a disruptor of the practice of healthcare but rather it augments the traditional delivery of healthcare and enables a more agile and continuous mechanism of care provision, which engages the patient more strongly as an equal partner in their care.

Telemedicine adoption has increased among clinicians and patients and we are now focused on promoting safe, effective, patient-centered, and equitable care. Telehealth promotes self-management, reduces medical errors, improves resource utilization and transitions cost savings to patients and their families. Each individual cardiology practice will find they have a range of provider adoption and use cases for blended virtual and in-person care. Across all practices however, establishing telemedicine workflows to ensure appropriateness of services, engagement in shared-decision making and promoting patient education and self-advocacy will be consistent themes.

A. B. Bhatt (✉)
Harvard Medical School, Boston, MA, USA

Massachusetts General Hospital, Boston, MA, USA
e-mail: abhatt@mgh.harvard.edu

S. Nagale
Digital Health & Data Services, Boston Scientific, Marlborough, MA, USA
e-mail: sandra.nagale@bsci.com

© Springer Nature Switzerland AG 2021
A. B. Bhatt (ed.), *Healthcare Information Technology for Cardiovascular Medicine*, Health Informatics, https://doi.org/10.1007/978-3-030-81030-6_1

1.1 Cardiovascular Healthcare Technology

Cardiology is the ideal discipline for the practice of telemedicine. As the infrastructure is built, it is essential to recognize that virtual and in-person care have a synergistic role, complementing one another to improve access and create safe, high quality care. Clinicians and patients must not expect a virtual visit to mirror a face to face visit, as it will have its own workflow as well as experience. Cardiologists need to be actively involved in the evaluation of digital medical technologies and administrators need to establish clear workflows to ease the transition to blended care by removing administrative barriers (Table 1.1). Lastly, reimbursement must be tied to patient satisfaction, provider reduction in burnout, quality of outcomes of care and adoption of new mechanisms of care delivery to truly establish a sustainable model of blended cardiac care delivery.

The consumer-electronics market is also driving patients towards more sophisticated telemedicine capable technology at home. Smartphones are capable of gathering bio-parameters and sensor data, with patients using smartphones for video visits, healthcare data collection, medical prompts and education. The familiarity of using one's phone to leverage a telemedicine monitoring platform to track their cardiovascular status carries value for the patients, doctors, hospitals and payers. Algorithms can then be taught to improve chronic care, and have already demonstrated improvements in medication adherence and blood pressure control [3]. Consumer purchased peripherals will continue to grow in number and purpose and produce aggregate data and the individual and community level (Fig. 1.1). A unique advantage of these peripherals is their ability to monitor health discreetly, thereby addressing health data collection with cultural sensitivity. As patients engage with providers remotely, they are increasingly engaged in, and can bring added benefit

Table 1.1 Technological capabilities

a. Audio
b. Text messaging, email
c. Chatbots
d. Patient portals for virtual check-ins (eg. MyChart)
e. Video 2-way: Apple FaceTime, Facebook Messenger Video Chat, Google Hangouts Video, Zoom, Skype
f. HIPAA compliant video technologies: Skype/MS Teams, Updox, VSee, Zoom for Healthcare, Doxy.me, Updox, Google G Suite Hangouts Meet, Cisco Webex Meetings, Amazon Chime, GoTo Meeting, Spruce Health Care Messenger, American Well, MD Live, BlueJeans for Healthcare, Doximity
g. Wearable devices and implantable devices (patient)
h. Surgery telementoring systems – InTouch, Avail, Proximie, ExplORer
i. Wearables/ Augmented reality: Video glasses (Google glass), MS Hololens
j. Automatic data upload (no need for patient to do anything before e-visit)
k. Adjacent integrated solutions eg. integrated scheduling and data collection/analytics, payment, insurance claims, etc. around telemedicine event

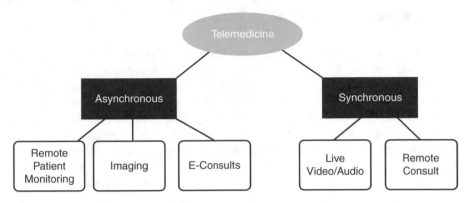

Fig. 1.1 Asynchronous vs. synchronous telemedicine

Table 1.2 Telemedicine needs by type of user

Non-surgical	
Clinical to patient	• Remote visits (follow-ups, refills & consultations • Remote patient monitoring (non-invasive devices, implanted devices) • Remote decision support, tele-triage • Remote pre-visit prep • Inpatient
Physician to caregiver/patient	• Virtual rounding • Remote video consult with family and clinician
Physician to physician	• Remote consult • Education/telemonitoring • Remote learning (clinician training) • Multidisciplinary team assessment
Surgical	
Physician to physician	• Surgical telementoring • Teleproctoring
Physician to patient	• Pre-operative screening • Post-operative follow-up • Post-discharge nursing follow up • Virtual cardiac rehab
Live cases/physician groups	• Remote live case education • Surgery broadcasting • Remote conferences

to, their local communities. Optimization of long term management in the community decreases chronic disease patient utilization of urgent care, and instead enables central institutions to focus on episodic emergent care, further improving resource utilization (Table 1.2). As sensors increase in number and with more disease specific value and via measurable RPM platforms, their financial value should soon be realized.

1.2 Impact of the COVID-19 Pandemic

Pre-COVID, telemedicine was available (through large provider networks and employers) but not widely adopted. It often did not cover small practices/local physicians but instead centered on programs implemented at large hospitals. Consumers were often unaware that their physicians offered telehealth services. [2] Other major reasons for not using telehealth were preference for in-person interaction, privacy concerns, perceived challenges with technology, or lack of access to broadband. Provider level barriers included uncertainty about reimbursement, provider-patient workflow, incorporation of technology and ability to provide high quality care. Fortunately, a recent Cochran review revealed similar outcomes between in-person and telephone visits for patients with chronic conditions (diabetes, CHF) [9]. Similarly, in a pilot of heart failure virtual visits, 108 patients transitioning from hospital to home revealed a lower no-show rate for virtual vs in-person visits and no significant difference in hospital readmissions, ER visits, and death [4].

During the COVID Pandemic, telemedicine evolved rapidly as an instrumental enabler of remote hospital practices during the COVID-19 digital revolution. The use of telemedicine and virtual visits were used to address essential needs for both COVID and non-COVID patients. In addition to remotely connecting with and treating those patients infected with COVID-19, it also provided the opportunity to see healthy patients virtually to limit exposure to and spread of the disease and enabled remote (quarantined) physicians to work. In the spring of 2020, there was a significant surge in telemedicine adoption from 8% to 90% virtual visits across all specialities in the United States [8] with a 135% increase in virtual urgent care and 4345% increase in non-urgent care delivery [6]. There was considerable flexibility offered to HIPAA-enabled healthcare institutions, offering HCPs permission to use remote communication technologies (Facetime, Facebook Messenger, Google Hangouts, Zoom, Skype) even if not yet HIPAA compliant. Simultaneously, many Medicare restrictions were lifted allowing providers to provide patient care remotely, across state lines, deliver care to new patients, and bill telehealth at a comparable level as for in-person services. Unfortunately, the fear during COVID-19 of presenting for in-person care did drive patients to remain silent with symptoms or delay seeking care, resulting in late, more severe cardiovascular disease progression with delayed urgent and emergent cardiovascular care.

Post-Covid, telemedicine is here to stay and will aid in the fast evolution of the "new healthcare practice". Telemedicine enables physicians and nurses to work remotely, delivering high quality care, and augmenting in-person traditional care [10]. With patients and providers now appreciating the ease of use and convenience of virtual care, regulatory changes implemented during pandemic enabling rapid telemedicine) might be difficult to reverse post-COVID [7].

1.3 Ensuring Equitable Care

As blended virtual and in-person encounters continue to be rapidly adopted for the longitudinal provision of outpatient cardiac care, ensuring the delivery of high quality, equitable care is essential. Phone visits during times like the COVID-19 pandemic are a useful mechanism to ensure communication between patient and clinician. However, for optimal, long term care, video visits offer clinicians the ability to see the patient in their environment, respond to facial cues (i.e. pain, emotion, and comprehension), use image sharing for education and data review, and perform a virtual physical exam. It also gives physicians the unique opportunity to simultaneously connect with the patient's family and caregivers. Cardiovascular management is also improved with vital sign monitoring and with integration into the EMR when possible. Navigating the use of new remote patient monitoring devices can also be taught during video visits. Therefore, it is essential to understand the barriers to video-based virtual care as well as the predictors of successful adoption (Table 1.3).

Telecardiology can promote timely intervention, access for those living in medically underserved areas, and increased access to specialists by increasing provider

Table 1.3 Telemedicine issues and risks

1. Learning curve for new technology	Need for training
2. Implementation of new hospital/clinic guidelines	Need for new reimbursement, payment policies and credentialing across hospitals
3. Need to quickly enable smaller hospitals with telehealth	They are at a disadvantage vs teaching hospitals w established programs but essential to provide care to patients remote from big cities/hospitals
4. Implementation of new security guidelines	Privacy, cybersecurity, interoperability, hospital reuse of technology
5. Legal, regulatory issues	Obtaining Class I/II FDA approval for telehealth solutions like eICU, telementoring, etc.
6. Technology hurdles for seniors	May not be using as much as younger or population. • 11–24% seniors have used telehealth in COVID period but ~68% have access to technology. • Opportunity to access patients through their caregivers • Prolonged stay-at-home order may lead to an increased use by seniors • Studies show that seniors will use telehealth if protocol applies to their condition, technology is easy to use and care is personalized (ref. 7)
7. Clinician preparedness	Physicians need to be ready for "virtual rapport building, empathy, "facilitated" physical exams, diagnosis, and counseling" (ref. 10)
8. Patient Satisfaction and Accessibility to Provider	Patient preference to see their own provider vs someone else

capacity. It is important that we pre-plan to address disparities in care ensuring that we do not worsen the digital divide and target increased access to specifically overcome barriers to care in at-risk populations. Wide scale implementation of telemedicine requires an infrastructure which addresses vulnerable populations including the elderly, those with limited digital or health literacy, individuals with decreased access, including rural or impoverished urban areas, limited English proficiency, racial/ethnic minorities, and those with low income or inadequate insurance.

In older adults, visual and hearing impairment, cognitive decline and challenges with dexterity are just some of the deterrents to the utilization of video and digital technology. Future iterations of telemedicine workflows will need to include technical accommodations for sight and hearing limitations as well as hospital-based technology support. The close involvement of caregivers, family members and community advocates in preparation for and during these televisits will negate a worsening digital divide for access to care in the elderly.

Digital and health literacy need to be addressed concomitantly with telemedicine implementation. Health literacy is a ubiquitous challenge throughout any healthcare system. Patients with chronic cardiovascular disease and social barriers to access are also those who feel digitally disengaged. They will benefit from digital skill assessment and ongoing support as the field of telemedicine evolves. Importantly, digital literacy is dependent not only upon skills but also the individual's confidence with technology and can be further complicated by low health literacy. To proactively engage in healthcare, patients need to be facile with accessing services and comprehending basic health information for healthcare delivery to positively affect outcomes.

Telemedicine offers an opportunity to address structural racism. Meeting the patient in their home provides a window into their environment and a chance to demonstrate respect and build trust with the individual and their family. Video visits enable us to tailor the patient's care based not only on medical diagnoses but also on their social determinants of health. While telemedicine eliminates physical barriers to the delivery of care, we must actively avoid infrastructures which create digital isolation as a new barrier to accessing healthcare. Nearly half of the US population has slow or unreliable internet connection which contributes to isolation and decreased health literacy. While national legislation is underway to improve digital access, local efforts can include free Wi-Fi in rural and urban at-risk settings as well as the use of text messaging to minimize the impact of video streaming on limited data plans. At the clinician level, in addition to implicit bias and cultural competency training, equity dashboards can aid in awareness of existing inequities to allow practices to directly address unmet needs.

Trust in the healthcare system becomes increasingly important as we increase the virtual and digital footprint of chronic disease management. Research confirms that Black patients are more likely to seek preventive care from Black physicians: racial concordance could reduce the cardiovascular mortality gap between black and white patients by nearly 20% [1]. It is our responsibility to seek out and train a diverse and culturally competent workforce as we educate the next generation and create digital health leaders. Our current systems must also be reviewed to ensure equitable distribution of virtual care and implement tools and programs to aid patients in advocating for themselves and their communities. However, it is certain that multifaceted interventions will be necessary to achieve equity and address the dynamic SDOH that affect access to care including insurance, education, housing, wealth, racism.

1.4 Quality Measures and Cost-Effectiveness in Telecardiology

In this book we will address the stakeholders essential to creating financially viable models for virtual care as well as the quality metrics needed to ensure safe and appropriate care delivery. While patients and providers are central to these processes, we will discuss the role of payers as essential stakeholders who impact the financial landscape of telemedicine through payment policies, benefit design, sales channels, government bid process, and, influence management of governmental insurance and medical coverage. There is a pivotal role for managing risk and cost in chronic disease populations by having care management teams help guide virtual vs. in-person care. Adopting the use of telemedicine will create cost savings where ordinarily unplanned utilization of care and ancillary authorization have created a financial burden. Improving access by expanding the geographic area of coverage and addressing social determinants of health can avert emergency utilization and brick and mortar overhead, thereby decreasing costs (16). In healthcare reimbursement models like those in the United States, payer quality is dependent on subjective feedback and the member's convenient access to care using telemedicine may favorably impact quality metrics. Although telemedicine initially replaced non-emergent medical care in response to the COVID-19 pandemic, as pandemic wanes, cardiologists the world over must demonstrate the continued advantage of blended in-person and virtual care for patients and payers alike.

1.5 Conclusion

Telemedicine rapid evolution post-COVID is driving fast adoption and imposing the demand for support of the new tools and support for larger scale. The choice of the right telemedicine technologies can help physicians, healthcare practitioners and patients recreate the future in-person experience; thereby creating an opportunity to reduce healthcare risks and create savings. In the future and for telemedicine to address the needs, it will be important to incorporate it within the rest of digital health solutions (devices, patient and physician software and applications, data analytics), maintain appropriate regulatory, privacy and security compliance within the application, and integrate telemedicine into existing clinical workflows (Fig. 1.2).

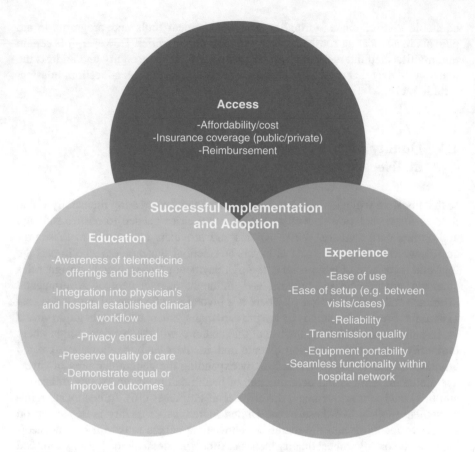

Fig. 1.2 Successful implementation and adoption

In this book we will explore the many facets of telecardiology including evaluating digital medical technologies, integrating wearables and remote patient monitoring and understanding the delegation of responsibility for data. We will also address the key mechanisms to build a digital heart center and explore the role of telemedicine as a growth strategy for improving patient experience, provider satisfaction and access to care. An emphasis of this book will be to alert readers to the risk of worsening the digital divide, and practical mechanisms to create structurally equitable virtual care paradigms. In an era of physician burn-out, improved engagement with telemedicine leads to opportunities for clinician creativity, productivity and higher quality care. Relationships are essential to the human connection and in a touching chapter on urgent care delivery, we will examine the positive effect of telemedicine on patient and provider engagement. Looking ahead, there is a need to consider our role in working with payers, developing curricula for virtual care delivery education and incorporating artificial intelligence to optimize care. Deliberate attention to these facets of telemedicine as we redesign cardiac care will create clinician-patient partnerships for longer, healthier lives.

1.6   Telemedicine Advantages

1. Keep patients out of hospital/ reduce ER visits
2. Bypassing ER visit, bypass prep, PCP exam, direct route for patient to hospital bed
3. Help enable social distancing compliance (non-urgent visits)
4. Enable combination of in-person and remote (quarantined) staff
5. Help physician with better-informed scheduling decisions for elective visits and surgeries
6. Better care for patients in rural areas
7. Enables better care for the elderly, disabled, unable to travel
8. Social determinants of health: telehealth an important vehicle for healthcare delivery for patients without housing and public transit
9. Physicians benefit from seeing patient in their home environment
10. Ability to 'bring along' caregiver for the visit
11. Opportunity for better harmonization and integration of patient data and clinical workflows through software solutions
12. Telemedicine may generate more meaningful data, leading to more insights, more future healthcare solutions
13. Faster decision making by care providers
14. Reduce number of visitors in hospitals
15. Enable remote visits to quarantined areas using telemedicine equipment
16. Easier for patients to discuss difficult topics and can have family presence during visit
17. Hospitals continue to generate revenue and able to reallocate resources
18. Ensure continuation of clinical/research studies
19. Reduce need for in-person physician interactions (procedure mentoring, proctoring, education, etc) via remote telemedicine equipment
20. Immediate access to specialized surgical expertise through telementoring, could have high impact to future patient care

1.7   Data and Analytics Enable Telemedicine

1. Data and algorithms for triaging (during COVID: travel history, exposure, vitals, other data)
2. Data obtained during tele-visit represent an opportunity to obtain more data *and* structured data when compared to an office visit
3. Opportunity for immediate data integration during digital visit
4. More data will be obtained due to video streaming, video capture during OR procedures - lead to more opportunity to educate others but also more privacy risk and need to ensure robust compliance

References

1. Alsan M, Stantcheva S, Yang D, Cutler D. Disparities in coronavirus 2019 reported incidence, knowledge, and behavior among US adults. JAMA Netw Open. 2020;3(6):e2012403.
2. CMS. Medicare telemedicine health care provider fact sheet. 2020. Retrieved 2020 Oct 9 from https://www.cms.gov/newsroom/fact-sheets/medicare-telemedicine-health-care-provider-fact-sheet
3. Fisher ND, Fera LE, Dunning JR, Desai S, Matta L, Liquori V, et al. Development of an entirely remote, non-physician led hypertension management program. Clin Cardiol. 2019;42(2):285–91.
4. Gorodeski E (2019. Virtual visits reduce no-show rates in heart failure patients. Retrieved from https://www.hcplive.com/view/virtual-visits-reduce-noshow-rates-in-heart-failure-patients
5. HHS. Telehealth: delivering care safely during COVID-19. 2020. https://www.hhs.gov/coronavirus/telehealth/index.html
6. Mann DM, Chen J, Chunara R, Testa PA, Nov O. COVID-19 transforms health care through telemedicine: evidence from the field. J Am Med Inform Assoc. 2020;27(7):1132–5. https://doi.org/10.1093/jamia/ocaa072. PMID: 32324855; PMCID: PMC7188161
7. Mann DM, Chen J, Chunara R, Testa PA, Nov O. COVID-19 transforms health care through telemedicine: evidence from the field. J Am Med Inform Assoc. 2020;
8. Mehrotra A, Chernew M, Linetsky D, Hatch H, & Cutler D. What impact has COVID-19 had on outpatient visits?. 2020. Retrieved from https://www.commonwealthfund.org/publications/2020/apr/impact-covid-19-outpatient-visits
9. Orozco-Beltran D, Sánchez-Molla M, Sanchez JJ, Mira JJ, ValCrònic Research Group. Telemedicine in primary care for patients with chronic conditions: the ValCrònic Quasi-Experimental Study. J Med Internet Res. 2017;19(12):e400.
10. TCTMD (2020). Telehealth offers a lifeline for cardiology patients during the COVID-19 pandemic. (https://www.tctmd.com/news/telehealth-offers-lifeline-cardiology-patients-during-covid-19-pandemic).

Further Reading

AMA quick guide to telemedicine in practice. https://www.ama-assn.org/practice-management/digital/ama-quick-guide-telemedicine-practice?gclid=CjwKCAjw5cL2BRASEiwAENqAPrIMl_VaG90-r36DJd5k1NQdM3MpX9I7vFahJPbzZCxT6ewaEMFg7xoCTxQQAvD_BwE and https://www.ama-assn.org/system/files/2020-04/ama-telehealth-playbook.pdf
COVID-19: the rise and rise of telemedicine. https://www.mobihealthnews.com/news/europe/covid-19-rise-and-rise-telemedicine
COVID-19 shifts Telehealth to the Center of Cardiology. https://www.medscape.com/viewarticle/927465
FAQs on Telehealth and HIPAA during the COVID-19 nationwide public health emergency. https://www.hhs.gov/sites/default/files/telehealth-faqs-508.pdf
https://pubmed.ncbi.nlm.nih.gov/32220575/
Surg Endosc. 2016;30:3665–72.
Surg Endosc. 2019;33:684–90.
Surveys suggest seniors aren't using telehealth during COVID-19 crisis. https://mhealthintelligence.com/news/surveys-suggest-seniors-arent-using-telehealth-during-covid-19-crisis
Telehealth coding and billing during COVID-19. https://www.acponline.org/practice-resources/covid-19-practice-management-resources/telehealth-coding-and-billing-during-covid-19
Telehealth: delivering care safely during COVID-19. https://www.hhs.gov/coronavirus/telehealth/index.html

Telehealth: rapid implementation for your Cardiology Clinic. https://www.acc.org/latest-in-cardiology/articles/2020/03/01/08/42/feature-telehealth-rapid-implementation-for-your-cardiology-clinic-coronavirus-disease-2019-covid-19

Telemedicine in the Era of COVID-19. Editorial. J Allergy Clin Immunol Pract. 2020 May. https://reader.elsevier.com/reader/sd/pii/S221321982030249X?token=E02C3738158B2FF2D4AE434B1421339B22D3EB0B1AA16F6FF1A2EBECCB68E67DBDCF7697D05FCFEF5E61644778360EC7

The evolution of surgical telementoring: current applications and future directions. Ann Transl Med. 2016;4(20):391. https://www.ncbi.nlm.nih.gov/pmc/articles/PMC5107399/pdf/atm-04-20-391.pdf

The role of telehealth in combating the social determinants of health. https://www.healthrecovery-solutions.com/blog/telehealth_sdoh

Virtual visits for care of patients with heart failure in the era of COVID-19: a statement from the Heart Failure Society of America. J Card Fail. 2020 Apr 18. https://www.ncbi.nlm.nih.gov/pmc/articles/PMC7166039/

Virtually perfect? Telemedicine for COVID-19. N Engl J Med. 2020;382:1679–81. https://www.nejm.org/doi/full/10.1056/NEJMp2003539

Chapter 2
Digital Health Solutions and Wearable Devices

Jennifer M. Joe, Jaydeo Kinikar, Monique Smith, Michael J. Carr, Ethan Bechtel, Stephen Randall, and Leah Ammerman

Digital health has been defined by the Healthcare Information and Management Systems Society (HIMSS) as "Digital health connects and empowers people and populations to manage health and wellness, augmented by accessible and supportive provider teams working within flexible, integrated, interoperable and digitally-enabled care environments that strategically leverage digital tools, technologies and services to transform care delivery" [1].

The original version of this chapter was revised. The correction to this chapter can be found at https://doi.org/10.1007/978-3-030-81030-6_11

J. M. Joe (✉)
Vanguard.Health, Boston, MA, USA
e-mail: jen@vanguard.health.com

J. Kinikar
VP, Virtual Care Offering Management, Best Buy Health, Boston, MA, USA

M. Smith
Health DesignED: The Acute Care Design and Innovation Center, Emory University School of Medicine, Atlanta, GA, USA
e-mail: monique.antoinette.smith@emory.edu

M. J. Carr
Emory University School of Medicine, Atlanta, GA, USA
e-mail: michael.j.carr@emory.edu

E. Bechtel
OhMD, Burlington, VT, USA
e-mail: ethan@ohmd.com

S. Randall
Medaica Inc., Brooklyn, NY, USA
e-mail: stephen.randall@medaica.com

L. Ammerman
IC Solutions & Partnerships, Boston Scientific, Boston, MA, USA
e-mail: Leah.Ammerman@bsci.com

© Springer Nature Switzerland AG 2021, corrected publication 2022   13
A. B. Bhatt (ed.), *Healthcare Information Technology for Cardiovascular Medicine*, Health Informatics, https://doi.org/10.1007/978-3-030-81030-6_2

Generally, digital health refers to technological solutions that go beyond the traditional electronic medical record. Important concepts that are frequently talked about are included in the table below (Table 2.1).

Most digital health solutions will typically involve 2–3 of these concepts. For example, a smart blood pressure monitor acts as a wearable device for the patient, which gathers data, stores it locally and transmits it via applications to the physician. Using algorithms, clinicians can assess populations of patients for blood pressure trends, highlighting those who are "out of range" to optimize medical therapy [2]. Eventually, increased sophistication in algorithms which receive clinician feedback and guidance can lead to the application of machine learning for hypertension management.

Table 2.1 Digital health overview

Wearables	The classic example that has become somewhat ubiquitous is the activity tracker watch that reports steps, distance, heart rate, calories and sleep quality. There are also headbands that will track concentration and even bras that monitor heart rhythms.
Sensors	For a wearable to be useful, they often have sensors attached to them that are doing the measuring. Due to the use of pulse oximetry monitors that are attached to a patient's finger on almost every clinical visit, the concept of a sensor attached to a wearable is very familiar. In healthcare, the quality of the sensor is important. New sensors enter the market daily, however, their accuracy for clinical decision making is often not proven.
Software Applications	This is the software, often in the form of a phone application, sometimes with a desktop version, that collects the data and displays it in a meaningful way. When done well, this data will do two important things—inform and change the patient's behavior for better health, and go to the clinical team so that this data can be incorporated into the patient's chart for the entire clinical team to use.
Data	Data is being gathered, stored, and shared. Important questions in healthcare is where the data is stored, who has access to the data, and is the data being delivered in a consistent and meaningful way? The biggest complaint in healthcare is "interoperability," or the simple concept of data moving from one source to another in a meaningful way. For example, if your watch collects three heart rates for you, how does the watch Iabel that data so that your electronic medical record can suck it in, and also label it in a meaningful way? A heart rate of 130 is appropriate If you're sprinting, and pathological if you're sleeping.
Big Data	This refers to a mass of data that informaticians are analyzing, interpreting, and looking for patterns. Informaticians will write algorithms to predict based on large collections of data, and this is referred to as artificial intelligence.
Augmented Reality	Augmented reality enhances reality or adds an overlay on top of what you're seeing and hearing in the environment. Google Glass is a classic example. It has a small screen that overlays on top of what you're seeing, possibly telling you the name of a building that you're looking at, or giving you directions with arrows overlaying the streets you are actually looking at.
Virtual Reality	Virtual reality is a much more immersive experience, requiring the technology to replace what you are seeing and hearing in reality. This is commonly delivered with a special VR headset. AR and VR haven't fully found homes within healthcare however, their most promising use-cases have been for pain control, meditation and surgical education.
Population Health	This is the use of big data, algorithms and software to help give clinicians an overview of the overall health of the population they are managing.

2.1 Clinicians as Digital Health Champions

Healthcare has been described as the "last frontier" of digital transformation in large part because of its complexity and heterogeneity [3]. Privacy issues may limit software developer's access to clinician expertise and intuition and if a solution fails, it can result in significant morbidity and even mortality.

A clinician will be best suited to influence the development of a digital solution that will be useful for their specific patient population. The practice of medicine is now highly subspecialized and influenced by prolific research. Clinicians also have considerable experience with particular diagnoses and their patients' unique psychosocial needs. Additionally, the clinician often has insight into the full care-team picture. For digital health to successfully infiltrate medicine, it needs clinicians as digital health champions. (Table 2.2).

2.1.1 Evaluating a Digital Solution

For a digital solution to be widely adopted, it must prove that it has a meaningful impact on care. This is often done as a randomized, clinical trial, however to move at the pace of current day digital health, clinicians will be essential to guiding widely accepted surrogate endpoints and definitive endpoints such as blood pressure measurements, adherence to guideline directed medical therapy and hospital admissions [4].

One of the biggest hurdles is making sure the digital health solution fits into the clinical environment and workflow. Due to compliance, the electronic medical record, payer requirements and billing requirements, healthcare seems like a huge mess of unnecessary paperwork and checkboxes. The digital health solution may fit into an already existing workflow, and preferably integrate into the electronic medical record [5].

For any digital health solution to work, it must have a clinician championing it's through the system [6]. It's often the clinician champion that will introduce the solution into their environment, get other stakeholder buy-in, and shepherd it through the process of information technology integration, security and legal compliance, testing on a small group, validation on a larger group, and then roll out at scale.

The clinician has an important role as the digital health advocate. They can guide the community on the benefits and the challenges they may encounter, guide

Table 2.2 The advantages of clinicians as digital health champions

1. Understand the problem to be solved
2. Know what patients need
3. Open to novel or creative solutions
4. Assess meaningful impact on care
5. Develop clinical workflow and promote telemedicine adoption

developers of solutions, including pharma, biotech, medical device manufacturers, non-traditional healthcare like Google and Amazon, as well as clinicians and hospital or practice managers and stakeholders.

2.2   Successfully Implementing a New Digital Health Solution

Many cardiovascular clinicians are approached and interested in working with new digital health solutions. However, the challenge is often in seeing the product which is offered and matching it to a need in your practice. At the same time, patient and provider adoption needs to be addressed in the early stages of development, whether via eliciting feedback, running "pilots", or acknowledging and solving for the most vexing care delivery problems. There are a few key steps which can help the new digital health clinician and administrator in selecting and templating a novel care mechanism or workflow (Fig. 2.1).

1. Quick Wins: Start with challenges which may be easiest to address. This offers a short-term, realistic attempt to implement a digital solution. This will garner patient, clinician and administrative trust in digital health solutions).
2. Cross the Finish Line: Iterate on problems with other solutions that have recently been tried. Multiple attempts to fix an existing flaw in care delivery demonstrates dedication to addressing the problem, while increasing the likelihood that stakeholders will be willing to try a novel digital solution if standard approaches have proven unsuccessful.
3. Measurable Endpoints: Working with the digital health team to scope the problem, this ensures that the issue to be addressed is well-defined and creates measurable endpoints for patient care (improved access, financial recovery, use of guideline directed medical therapy). After each iteration of a solution, clinical team feedback is key to growth and improvement. Once a "final model" is in place, testing and validation should be part of the overall plan with the digital health company. It is important to recognize that creating a solution, which is

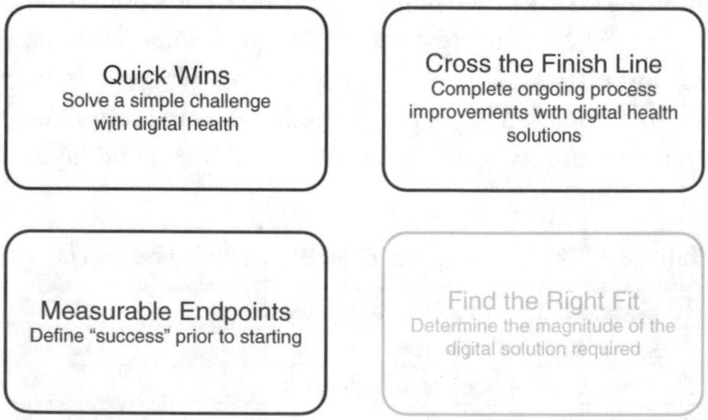

Fig. 2.1 Successful implementation of a new digital health solution

Quick Wins
Solve a simple challenge with digital health

Cross the Finish Line
Complete ongoing process improvements with digital health solutions

Measurable Endpoints
Define "success" prior to starting

Find the Right Fit
Determine the magnitude of the digital solution required

modular from the beginning can allow for faster updates as clinical needs and workflow evolve in the practice.

4. Find the Right Fit: Some problems require small tech solutions while others need a well-established digital platform or system-wide implementation. There are advantages to small tech providers and larger firms. Small providers can be nimble and responsive to your needs and changes whereas larger providers may be more reliable long term. Assessing the importance of integration and consumer (both patient and clinician) support are both essential in evaluating digital health solutions and vary across novel and established platforms.

Evaluating a digital solution requires understanding the exact problems that need to be solved or the part of the workflow that is best treated virtually. Once a practice builds their digital solution, larger scale adoption may necessitate partnering with community organizations, pharmaceutical, device and technology companies. Successful implementation requires buy-in from administration, providers and patients with a clear alignment and understanding of the goals of using virtual care in addition to traditional in-person visits.

2.3 Wearable Devices

Telemedicine has become a mainstay of outpatient care. Patient level data, often obtained using wearables will likely play a role as patient adoption increases. These digital health tools abound is a necessity to scale telemedicine use and may improve access to advanced cardiac care (Fig. 2.2). In this chapter, we will explore considerations for designing clinically relevant wearables and measuring their value (Fig. 2.3). Determining the future of wearables will require engagement of patients, clinicians and industry (Fig. 2.4).

2.3.1 Wearables: Considerations for Designing Wearables Strategy Across the Patient Journey

Essential to the successful integration of digital health into any telemedicine system, is understanding the clinical, operational and financial goals of technology implementation (Table 2.3). Clear definition of the intended effect of digital health will enable staff workflow, promote patient and provider adoption and engender support from leadership.

The adoption of wearable devices is dependent primarily on ease of use, wireless accessibility and potential patient health benefits. Familiarity with the device that is being used as well as clinician recommendation can be catalysts for patient adoption (Table 2.4).

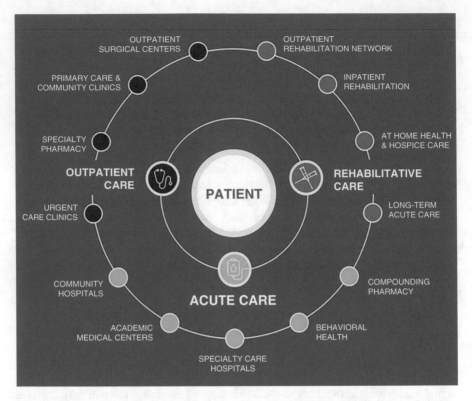

Fig. 2.2 Using telemedicine throughout the inpatient to outpatient cycle to reduce readmissions and increase convenience and quality of care. (From MGB Quality and Safety. Copyright permission from Mass General Brigham)

2.3.2 New Technologies: Integrating and Measuring to Deliver Value

Choosing the right digital health technology is only half the battle. Rest of the battle lies in generating buy-in from your key stakeholders for adoption and then driving continuous value realization to ensure you are getting ROI and continued investment support.

A holistic framework to integrate and measure value is through **Quadruple Aim** (Fig. 2.5).

The goal of the Quadruple Aim is to enhance patient experience, improve population health, reduce costs, and improve the work life of health care providers, including clinicians and staff. The Quadruple Aim is widely accepted as a compass to optimize health system performance. If you can link the value of your digital health initiative to one or more pillars of Quadruple Aim, you can then articulate the impact and ROI on KPIs that matter most to your stakeholders- administrators, clinicians and patients.

Fig. 2.3 Integrating telemedicine into clinical workflow based upon technological compatibility and clinical evidence

Workflow Integration

How seamless is data transfer and integration with informatics platform? How frequently is data collected? More continuous for hospital applications while every few min to every hour for home long term RPM. Does it require custom integration, or it supports standard interoperability such as HL7 feed? And how is wearables vital sign data validated in EMR?

Connectivty & Compatibility

How is data transferred from the wearable to EMR/informatics platform? Is it Bluetooth? WiFi? 5G? what is the hub/relay/bridge that provides connectivity? Is it 1:1 or 1: many? How does this hub fit into existing IT infrastructure? What about home? How easy is it to configure and connect at home for elderly at risk patient?

Is it compatible with other monitoring devices or does it cause interference? Is it compatible with pacemakers and implantable defibrillators?

Clinical Evidence

What clinical proof points are availble for this wearables solution? Has it been sufficiently tested in clinical environment? What evidence is available for clinical, operational and financial outcomes in a proper end-to-end clinical study?

2.3.2.1 Value Pillar 1: Improving Clinician Experience

Physician burnout is affecting the majority of physicians today and results in huge cost to the organization. Several healthcare systems have implemented telehealth programs in the ED to reduce patient wait times and help clinicians better manage patients. Similarly, there are new digital health technologies that automate certain workflows and reduce nursing workload, which in turn drive better adoption. With every digital health technology, the usability, product interactions and E2E user experience can make a big difference in improving clinician experience over old care paradigms. So think about how your digital health technology is improving clinician experience, how can you quantify it?

Fig. 2.4 Using
telemedicine to enhance
patient experience,
clinician experience and
clinical performance

Patient Experience

How is the wear experience on frail skin? Does it cause skin
rash? Has wearable adhesive been tested for
biocompatibility? Can patient shower with the wearable?
Does it require disturbing patient frequently or at night to
take measurements? Does it provide mobility and freedom
of ambulation?

Clinician Experience

How long does it take to onboard patient on new wearable
including association, calibration & pairing? How does it fit
into existing clinical/nursing workflows? Does it reduce
workload during rounding or create more nursing burden?

Clinical Performance

- In general, not all wearables are equal when it comes
  to clinical accuracy & performance, even after getting
  required regulatory approval. Evaluate stated accuracy
  & performance of key parameters-is it accurate &
  precise enough to replace mandated vital sign
  measurement as a standard care (e.g, HR) ? or is it
  good enough to provide accurate enough trending
  information to aid in early detection of an adverse
  event (e.g, BP measurements)
- What do claims and indications say? Does it provide
  ambulatory measurements? Sensitivity to ambulation
  can provide wrong measurements and false alarms
- For cardiac patients, difference between single lead to
  multi-lead ECG wearable could be significant. However,
  it goes back to what problems you are trying to solve in
  which care setting. Post-op cardiac patient will require
  proper Telemetry vs diagnostic arrhythmia detection at
- wearable patch.

2.3.2.2 Value Pillar 2: Better Outcomes

Every organization measures and reports key outcomes on a regular basis. This creates several opportunities for digital health technologies to drive impact and adoption. There are clear KPIs such readmissions, length of stay, # of code blues, etc.
that could be measured and improved. For example, the VA has reduced readmissions significantly with a combination of telehealth and remote patient monitoring.

Table 2.3 What *clinical, operational and financial* problems are you trying to solve?

Hospital	Home

• **Clinical:**
  – Post-op patient monitoring/PACU, discharge readiness, early detection of deterioration in General Ward/Step down unit, preventing code blues and ICU throwback, reducing falls, cardiac patient monitoring
  – Target patient populations: Cardiac (CHF, MI, arrhythmias, BP), Diabetes (ulcer, infections), Respiratory (COVID-19, COPD, P.E. emphysema, Sepsis), Neurological, Post-Op (Knee and hip surgery)
• **Operational:**
  – Seamless transitions, workflow/rounding efficiency, low nurse: patient ratio, risk stratification, alarm fatigue, patient and staff satisfaction, lack of PPE, HAI concerns
• **Financial:**
  – Length of stay, ICU throwbacks, limited ICU bed capacity, revenue and margin
	• **Clinical:**
	  – At-risk population, Readmission within first week and 30–60–90 days
	  – Chronic disease management for long term (COPD, CHF, Arrhythmia, Hypertension, Diabetes)
	  – Infectious disease quarantine
	• **Operational:**
	  – Lack of real-time visibility into patient's health
	  – Emergency services vs early prediction of adverse events
	  – Limited Home Health Agency support
	• **Financial:**
	  – Readmission penalties
	  – Costly intervention/EMS
	  – Value based Care penalties

Table 2.4 Future opportunities for wearables and digital health tech

Emerging	• Smartphone, wearable-based sensors • Ingestible sensors	• Manual and automatic biometric data collection • Automatic biometric data collection	• Monitoring heart rate, steps, food intake, etc. • Digestible pill for tracking medication adherence
Experimental	• Artificial intelligence and machine learning • Virtual and augmented reality	• Diagnosis and treatment recommendations • Simulated therapy	• Imaging interpretations • Chat bot for mental health • Provider training • Tele-rehabilitation

2.3.2.3 Value Pillar 3: Lower Costs

There are tremendous cost savings that could be achieved by digital health. For example, the cost of undetected patient deterioration could result in loss of millions of dollars due to readmissions and penalties. Wearables and remote patient monitoring can help detect patient decompensation early and help potentially costly code blues and readmissions with proper early interventions. What are the cost levers that your digital technology can impact? Where do you see the most impact?

Fig. 2.5 Quadruple aim.
Source: https://digital.ahrq.
gov/acts/quadruple-aim

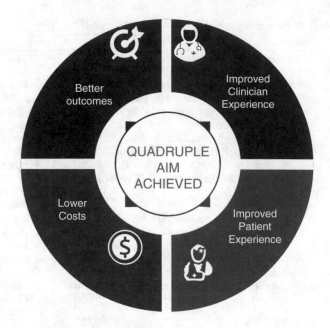

2.3.2.4 Value Pillar 4: Improved Patient Experience

Patient centric innovation helps improve patient experience, outcomes and adoption. It is also one of the key quality metrics that healthcare organizations measure and improve upon. A key imperative of digital health technology needs to be improving patient experience. It could be telehealth reducing wait times for patients or wearables providing freedom of movement in the hospitals or remote data collection from the comfort of their homes. How is your technology helping patients deal with their condition? How is it helping to normalize their lives?

2.4 Conclusion

Wearables hold significant promise for being a useful adjunct to cardiac outpatient management by allowing continuous data input for analysis of baselines and trends. They also offer opportunities for patient engagement, self-advocacy and goal setting. For digital health technologies to permeate clinical care across all populations there are several features which should be met. Ease of use with a natural daily instinct to include the wearable in their daily routine. Simple instructions to overcome limitations of digital and health literacy. Instruction available in text and with diagrams, but also online via audio and video to adapt to all learning styles for optimal understanding of its use. These mechanisms will aid those with visual, hearing or learning impairment by having accessible options for engagement, and ease the burden on clinical practices who can direct patients to this information. Minimizing the steps needed to transmit data is also essential with an ideal goal of automated data transmission.

Case Report

Leveraging an internal innovation center, Health DesignED: the Emory Acute Care Design and Innovation Center to tackle the special technical needs of the Emory Rural Tele-EMS Network (ER-TEMS) [8].

Physician Leaders: Monique Smith, MSc, MD, Founding Director of the Emory Acute Care Design + Innovation Center and Michael J. Carr, MD, Project director and Principle investigator ER-TEMS.

The COVID-19 pandemic has highlighted and intensified the increasing disparity in healthcare throughout the United States, which is particularly notable in underserved communities. One such community, which composes almost 20% (approximately 60 million people) of the population of the United States, are residents of rural communities. In 2019, the CDC reported that "Rural populations experience substantial health disparities when compared with more urban populations, including a higher prevalence of diseases such as obesity, increased mortality rates, and lower life expectancies."[9] Contributing significantly to this disparity in a community that is on average already sicker are the more than 120 rural hospitals—seven of which were in Georgia, that have closed in the United States in the last 10 years and the alarming 453 rural hospitals that are at risk of closing based upon performance levels [10]. This in turn, increases the time to care for patients by prolonging EMS response and transport times, which leads to poorer outcomes.

In a response to this, Emory has recently created the Emory Rural Tele-EMS Network to enhance timely diagnosis and treatment for rural Georgia patients. Emory physicians will provide clinical support to Grady EMS rural service providers. Currently, Grady EMS provides EMS services in 14 rural counties of Georgia. During an EMS encounter, critical patients will have a comprehensive telehealth visit with a physician to assess for pathology including cardiac arrest and arrhythmias, acute coronary syndromes, acute strokes, major trauma, labor and delivery emergencies, and hypertensive disorders. Once diagnosed, EMS personnel can provide care onsite, ultimately shortening time to the initiation of care, and subsequently transport the patient to the most suitable rural healthcare facility.

Although telehealth has become an increasingly accessible form of care, it is often not used in the prehospital environment and even less in rural areas. In rural environments where care delivery centers are scarce, the use of telehealth visits during EMS encounters has tremendous potential to change the EMS delivery model.

One of the few models of prehospital telehealth visits was initiated by Houston's Fire Department in 2014. The Emergency Telehealth and Navigation (ETHAN) program assessed and dispositioned patients using telehealth visits prior to transport to the appropriate care level e.g. Emergency Department (ED). The result of this initiative was a 56% reduction in unnecessary ambulance ED visits and 44 min reduction in total ambulance "back-in-service" times [11]. Overall, the researchers of the ETHAN program determined that these changes converted to $928,000 of societal annual cost savings and $2468 cost saving per ED visits averted [12].

Under the ER-TEMS network, an Emory Healthcare Network Emergency Physician provides a video telehealth visit to rural Grady EMS crews and evaluates and suggests management of initial patient care. If specialized care is needed, the Emergency Provider may access the vast network of specialty services within the Emory Healthcare Network. Subsequent to the consultation, all patient data, including biometric data, EKGs, and patient charts are uploaded to a streaming cloud. The Emergency Provider then informs the receiving facility, typically a critical access hospital (CAH) or hospital in a medically underserved area (MUA), of the incoming patient's arrival and any treatment plans that have been started. This allows EMS personnel to focus all of their attention on the patient's care. The receiving facility is given access to the cloud over the internet providing access to patient information and biometric data.

Prior to the Emory Rural Tele-EMS initiative, Emory had a robust telehealth network in multiple specialties, including the ICU, nephrology, and neurology and psychiatry starting as early as 2014. This network has accelerated and expanded rapidly in response to the COVID-19 pandemic. In the Spring of 2020, Emory Healthcare had successfully completed over 70,000 virtual visits. The pivot to telehealth prominence has been afforded by Medicare's 1135 waiver expansion, which allows telemedicine visits to be charged at the same rate as in-person emergency visits.

Despite Emory's considerable telemedicine experience, the Emory Rural Tele-EMS has radically different technological requirements. Firstly, Rural Tele-EMS needed a platform that would work both inside and outside the hospital. Secondly, the platform had to work in low bandwidth settings given the rural environment in which care would take place. To address this, the Emory Acute Care Design and Innovation Center was responsible for pinpointing, assessing, and testing solutions. A team was delegated to identify and evaluate solutions from Philips®, Zoll®, Verizon®, Stryker®, and swyMed® corporations.

Ultimately, Emory decided on swyMed, [13] which owns a patent on moving data in resource low settings and allows Emory to conduct telemedicine visits with transmission as low as 60 kilobits per second (kbps). This significantly increases the geographic reach of telemedicine utilization. Additionally, the Emory Acute Care Design and Innovation Center found it paramount that the telemedicine platform be able to integrate into EMS specific technology. SwyMed is integrated with Zoll—the X-series monitor/defibrillator used on Grady ambulances, hospital electronic medical record systems, and a number of other relevant medical devices and applications. This integration allows streaming directly from the Zoll-X monitor into the telemedicine interface, which can then be viewed on a desktop computer, or an app on a smartphone or tablet. The Zoll-X monitor has functionality that allows automatic streaming of the X-series data to the physician on the far-side of the video call while staying in the video call through just a press of a button. The swyMed interface is also HIPAA-compliant and encrypts the connection between the physician, ambulance, and the receiving hospital.

Furthermore, connectivity in rural settings requires special consideration. Thus, it was important for the Emory Acute Care Design and Innovation Center to identify the best data connectivity infrastructure. In Georgia, Verizon has the dominant cellular infrastructure. Resultantly, the Emory Acute Care Design and innovation Center's team contacted Verizon and confirmed that both Emory and swyMed could work with the Verizon network. Together, Emory and Verizon identified the AirLink MG-90 router (Sierra Wireless®, Vancouver, Canada) as the optimal solution. The AirLink MG90 offers up to 600 Mbps downlink and 150 Mbps uplink speeds over LTE Advanced Pro, 1.3 Gbps over dual radio, dual concurrent 3x3 MIMO 802.11 ac Wi-Fi, and 5-port Gigabit Ethernet. Grady EMS upgraded their entire system to use the AirLink MG-90 routers. Additionally, they created a list of ambulances that don't use the AirLink MG-90 router, and a plan and budget to install the needed AirLink MG-90 router.

This case report underscores that different technological requirements exist for different environments in which telemedicine takes place. Despite the existence of a robust telemedicine platform within the Emory Healthcare Network, this massive initiative was only made possible by having a dedicated internal innovation center, the Emory Acute Care Design and Innovation Center, to meaningfully and quickly roll out a complicated new care delivery system (Fig. 2.6).

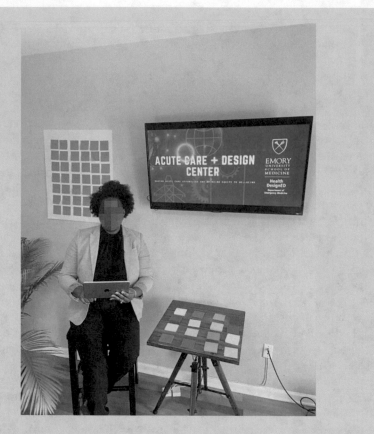

Used with Permission of Emory Department of Emergency Medicine.

Case Report: Remote Clinical Exam MEDAICA

Introduction

Medaica is a digital health company extending the capability of remote exams over any telehealth system, simply and affordably. The Company's first product is a consumer-focused digital stethoscope, designed specifically for telehealth systems at a price point that opens up the power and potential of remote care to all users. Medaica was founded by serial entrepreneurs with proven global experience in MedTech, Healthcare, Consumer Electronics and scaling mass volume hardware and software platforms.

The Problem

Existing telehealth systems provide video conferencing and/or chat applications, some with scheduling management and Electronic Medical Record (EMR) integration. Although telehealth is becoming increasingly popular, especially in light of COVID-19, it is currently limited to only a few practice areas, such as mental health, dermatology, pediatrics and the common cold. Auscultation is an important part of a clinical exam that is missing in telemedicine sessions. Addressing that need, not only has the potential to improve the effectiveness of remote care for both the clinician and patient, but also improve the utility and value of telehealth.

Medaica conducted extensive market research to surface the less obvious challenges of developing a product that required some level of behavioral change—both from doctors and consumers. Related to the introduction of blood pressure devices, pulse oximeters and, more recently, devices like the Kardia EKG, where patients use tools previously available only to clinicians, Medaica understood that clinicians AND patients need to recognize and want more valuable telemedicine sessions through such devices. The question was, would this be an acceptable proposition for both sides of the equation?

Insights

The Medaica design team (based in the USA and UK) spoke with many clinicians and received consistent feedback that most electronic stethoscopes are too complicated and too expensive for daily use. Furthermore, most electronic stethoscopes cleared by the FDA for use by clinicians, are NOT cleared for use by a "lay person" and, in a telemedicine session, it would be the patient, not the doctor, using the device.

Medaica also interviewed medical IT staff who are often the ones tasked with "making it work." IT professionals don't see the "wow" of a new device first but see the increased workload it might present. Incumbent proprietary solutions can create workflow silos that become increasingly difficult to manage and support. Solution providers need to understand and appreciate the time-consuming process of integrating IT services, devices and systems, and must not assume a doctor, clinic, or hospital will willingly adopt yet another proprietary solution. If every medical device only works with a specific telehealth platform, those devices ultimately become unsupported islands. That is not a sustainable strategy for a business or a medical practice.

At a detailed level, on top of familiar "hot button" issues including but not limited to data privacy and development of more telehealth pay-codes etc., examples of the less obvious but real-world challenges facing clinicians that also surfaced were:

- Artificial Intelligence AI, even when positioned as "Assisted Intelligence" which is arguably a friendlier and more accurate term of art, was often received as a threat not a benefit; At best it was a partial solution. For example, if a company offered an electronic stethoscope with AI that helps diagnose atrial fibrillation, the clinician still needed other devices, tests and protocols to diagnose other conditions such as arrhythmias, congenital heart disease, coronary artery disease, cardiomyopathy etc.

- Besides often generating a myriad of pairing issues, connecting a Bluetooth stethoscope during a telehealth session resulted in that device taking over the audio channel and the clinician being unable to talk with the patient.
- Devices that might not function before or during an exam because the battery was drained.
- Single purpose devices that often cost several hundred dollars were deemed not economically viable for a scalable solution and therefore did not warrant the time investment on the clinician's side to evaluate and/or integrate.

The resulting Venn diagram that became Medaica's mantra, was for its solutions to be; Affordable, Simple and Interoperable.

The Solution

Among Medaica's many different design decisions was their choice of using a USB cable (with adaptors for any laptop, desktop or mobile device) rather than Bluetooth. That simplified the electronic design and user experience, reduced the cost, avoided potential interference issues and removed the need for batteries. As a USB device, the Medaica stethoscope is "plug and play" and in its simplest form can securely send audio files, together with an "auscultation map" to the clinician either in store and forward or live modes.

The product design went through a number of iterations. It needed to be easy to hold but also easy to position in relation to the patient being able to position the device on an "auscultation map" in self-exam mode. One of the early designs was essentially a stethoscope head but was rejected because the user's hand would be covering the head and/or made a simple button push awkward (see Figs. 2.7 and 2.8).

The chosen design direction was to be more recognizably a stethoscope (see Fig. 2.9). The head of the device is easy to see (or detect for assisted positioning approaches) when the user is placing the device in a specific auscultation position. The design is easy to manufacture and can be completely sealed and therefore also has the advantage that it is washable to IP6X standards. These decisions were made prior to COVID-19 flaring up but become even more compelling within that context.

There were many technology decisions not only aimed at making the device easy to use, but easy to deploy and to potentially establish standard telehealth methods for patients and clinicians to quickly and easily share auscultation sounds. One of those decisions was to use two microphones configured for plug and play with any telehealth system, enabling both auscultation sounds and an independent channel for the user to speak, which also doubles for ambient/room noise reduction.

Because Medaica's solutions are designed to enhance existing telehealth solutions, not compete with them, they worked extremely hard to make sure that the clinician could continue to use whatever system they were already using, with the added benefit of adding auscultation to the exam. The pillars of that process were:

- Balance clinician AND patient ease of use to get a more valuable and informed telehealth consultation for both sides.
- Enable healthcare professionals to leverage existing workflows and systems.
- Don't compete with telehealth platforms—provide plug and play, agnostic, interoperability to any telehealth platform. Enable value-add to open their platforms to new specialties and stickier users.
- KISS (Keep It Simple Solutions)—solutions that work in the minimum number of steps with minimal behavioral change.
- Affordable—solutions that are priced for consumer scale.

OhMD Case Report

In the spring of 2020, the healthcare industry was rocked by the novel coronavirus disease (COVID-19). Almost overnight, HIPAA-compliant telehealth became a necessity for healthcare providers across the United States. Software companies everywhere raced to meet the demand. Among them was OhMD, a HIPAA-compliant texting platform that saw an obvious opportunity for growth.

When OhMD first launched video visits in early 2020, they expected it to be the clear solution to the sudden demand for telehealth. Providers quickly signed up for the new feature so they could continue working when social distancing measures went into place. While the video tool offered an essential alternative to in-person visits, there were obvious gaps in the new workflow. One practice that approached OhMD about the shortfalls was The Heart Medical Group in Van Nuys, CA. Providers wondered how to coordinate with patients to get them on the video call at the right time, and how to continue the conversation around treatment, payment and follow-up once they both clicked "end call". Essentially they needed to recreate the full in-office workflow of a patient visit, from check-in to intake to provider, and back to check-out.

To meet this need, OhMD was able to fall back on its core competency -- text messaging. With the addition of video visits, OhMD could now prompt a video visit appointment as a substitute for sitting down with a provider in the exam room and use secure texting to enable the rest of the practice workflow:

- The day before the visit (or anytime prior, in the case of same-day appointments), the care team texts the patient an appointment reminder and includes any forms that the patient needs to complete prior to the appointment. The patient taps the link to fill and submit the forms from their smartphone.

- Immediately before the appointment, the provider texts the patient to confirm they're ready. They send the patient a link which they tap to begin the video visit.
- When the call ends, the timestamps are stored in the patient thread for billing reference.
- The patient can then be reassigned in OhMD to administrative staff who handle payment through texted links, schedule necessary follow-up, and even request reviews.

The benefits of a sound telehealth strategy are of particular benefit to cardiologists and other specialties that deal with chronic illness. Some of the benefits to The Heart Medical Group include:

- OhMD allows patients who use remote patient monitoring (RPM) devices to text their provider with real time data on their health so they can make timely, appropriate recommendations on a patient's care.
- The ease and immediacy of texting strengthens the patient-provider relationship and improves patient adherence to care plans. Using a familiar, palatable channel like texting gives patients access to healthcare regardless of their fluency with technology.
- Telemedicine offers cost-saving benefits. Communication through texting helps patients save money on co-pays by reducing trips to the office. The effective deployment of telemedicine can also produce systematic savings by better triaging patients in lower acuity healthcare settings, reducing costly hospitalizations.
- Leveraging a platform like OhMD allows doctors to better allocate their time. Doctors can reduce unnecessary office visits, quickly and easily facilitate necessary visits, and improve chronic care management. This allows doctors to deliver the highest quality of care while focusing on revenue generation.

Cardiologists have found great success using OhMD for mixed telemedicine: a combination of traditional in-person care, virtual video visits, and two-way patient texting. OhMD has seen the incorporation of telemedicine increase provider capacity and accessibility, continuity of care, and overall quality of care. Although many providers viewed have adopted telehealth solutions as a short-term solution to care delivery during the COVID-19 pandemic, it has become clear that it adds indelible value to the healthcare system (Fig. 2.10).

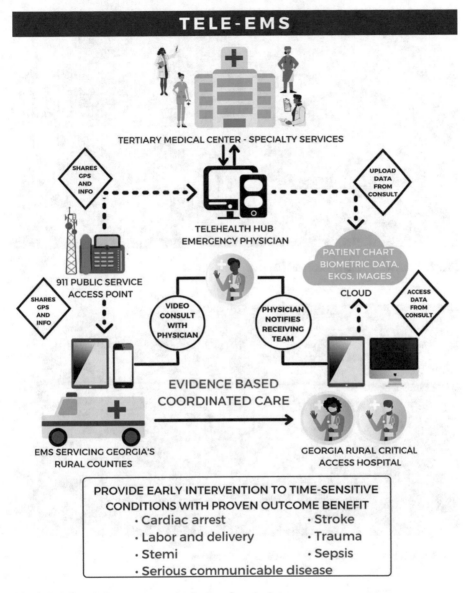

Fig. 2.6 Telemedicine emergency medical service triaging

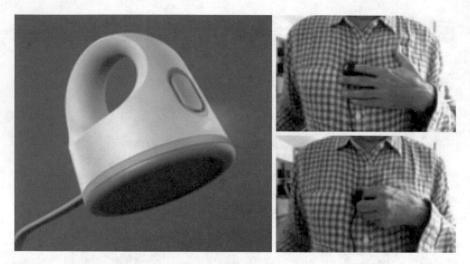

Fig. 2.7 Awkward button placement (*thumb*)

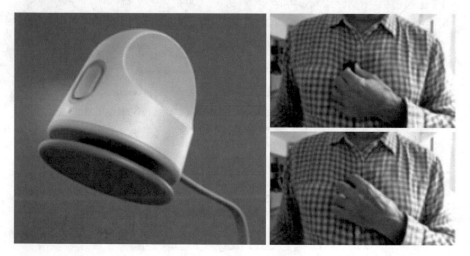

Fig. 2.8 OK button placement, but obscures head position

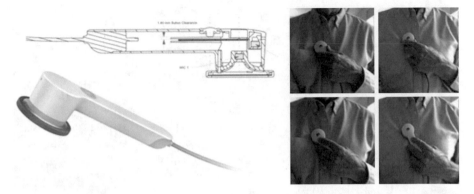

Fig. 2.9 Good button placement, good visibility of head position, comfortable to hold and separate body/voice mics

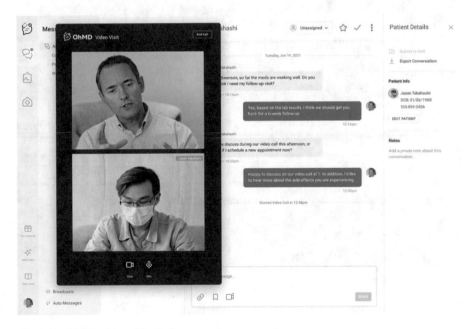

Fig. 2.10 OhMD video visit platform sample

Case Study: ASK ANGIE™

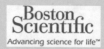

PCI procedures and devices are complex. There are times (day or night) when questions arise. ASK ANGIE is a technology provided by Boston Scientific that uses merged reality to instantly bring clinical expertise to the cath lab so that teams can confidently and efficiently perform complex cases, without delays, to deliver the best patient care. The merged reality functionality of ASK ANGIE allows certified Boston Scientific clinical representatives to give step-by-step guidance visually – as if they are in the cath lab in person. Clinicians can also use the tool to connect with their peers. In addition to merged reality calling, ASK ANGIE provides on-demand education that can help bring new lab staff up to speed or refresh tenured staff on procedures and technologies. ASK ANGIE delivers virtual support from expert reps for complex PCI devices and procedures.

The solution was initially piloted for 6 months, at remote facilities, with the help of clinician champions. The clinician champions saw the value and potential of the technology to meet their needs and helped work through the approval process to pilot the technologies with key stakeholders at their facility. We showed proof of concept through our minimum viable product (MVP) which supported ANGIOJET, a mechanical thrombectomy device. This tool is commonly used for emergency treatment of blocked arteries and thus cath lab staff frequently ask for support with device setup with little notice. To measure success, we looked at app usage and number of cases supported remotely. By selecting the right technology up front during the pilot, we were able to generate quick wins to fuel future innovation and maximize the potential for usage and adoption of the technology. After receiving feedback from users during initial pilots, we expanded the product scope to include

additional technologies. Eventually, we found the right fit by delivering educational content that supported all Complex PCI procedures, not just
thrombectomy.

It is important not to be wedded to any preconceived assumptions when
rolling out a new digital health technology. We initially thought only remote
facilities would be interested in ASK ANGIE. During the pilot we learned that
clinicians at larger facilities and in metropolitan areas found just as much
value in the technology as remote facilities. COVID-19 has expanded the
need and use case for this technology with facilities across the globe.

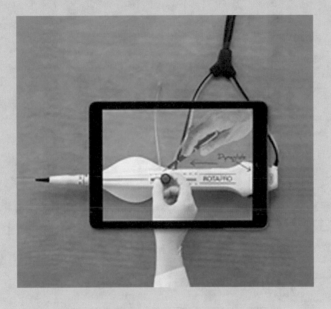

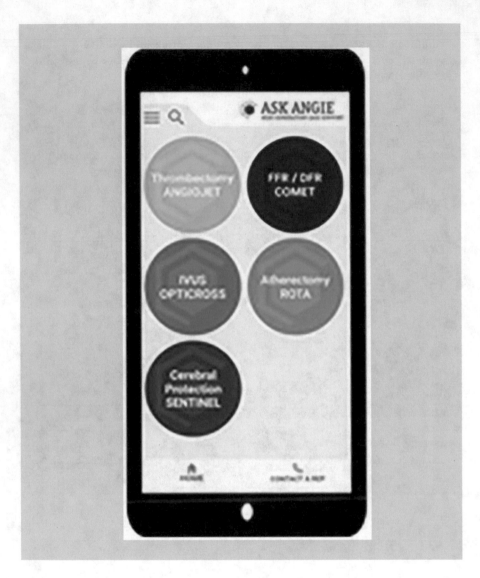

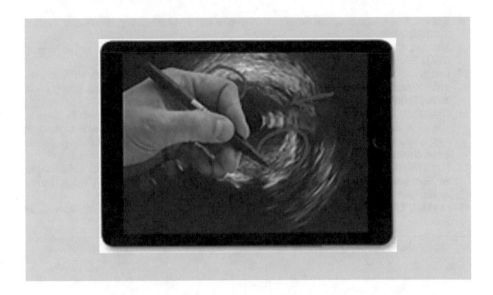

Acknowledgement   The Emory Rural Tele-EMS Network is supported by the Health Resources and Services Administration (HRSA) of the U.S. Department of Health and Human Services (HHS) as part of a financial assistance award totaling $1.2 million with 100 percentage funded by HRSA/HHS and zero percentage funded by non government source(s). The contents are those of Emory University and do not necessarily represent the official views of, nor an endorsement, by HRSA/HHS, or the U.S. Government.

References

1. Snowdon, A. (2020) Digital health.
2. Fisher ND, Fera LE, Dunning JR, Desai S, Matta L, Liquori V, et al. Development of an entirely remote, non-physician led hypertension management program. Clin Cardiol. 2019;42(2):285–91.
3. Staib A, Sullivan C, Prins JB, Burton-Jones A, Fitzgerald G, Scott I. Uniting emergency and inpatient clinicians across the ED–inpatient interface: the last frontier? Emerg Med Australas. 2017;29(6):740–5.
4. Guo C, Ashrafian H, Ghafur S, Fontana G, Gardner C, Prime M. Challenges for the evaluation of digital health solutions—a call for innovative evidence generation approaches. NPJ Digit Med. 2020;3(1):1–14.
5. Garg S, Williams NL, Ip A, Dicker AP. Clinical integration of digital solutions in health care: an overview of the current landscape of digital technologies in cancer care. JCO Clin Cancer Infor. 2018;2:1–9.
6. Van Velthoven MH, Cordon C. Sustainable adoption of digital health innovations: perspectives from a stakeholder workshop. J Med Internet Res. 2019;21(3):e11922.
7. Malec B. Healthcare information and management systems society 2016. J Health Adm Educ. 2016;33(4):625.

8. Estes C. 1 In 4 rural hospitals are at risk of closure and the problem is getting worse. Forbes. 2020 Feb 24;

9. James R, Champagne-Langabeer T, et al. Cost-benefit analysis of telehealth in pre-hospital care. J Telemed Telecare. 2017;23(8):747–51.

10. Langabeer JR, Gonzalez M, et al. Telehealth-enabled emergency medical services program reduces ambulance transport to urban emergency departments. West J Emerg Med. 2016;17(6):713–20.

11. Garcia MC, Rossen LM, Bastian B, Faul M, Dowling NF, Thomas CC, Schieb L, Hong Y, Yoon PW, Iademarco MF. Potentially excess deaths from the five leading causes of death in metropolitan and nonmetropolitan counties—United States, 2010–2017. CDC Surveillance Summaries. 2019. p. 1–11.

12. Sierra Wireless. AirLink® MG90/MG90 5G high performance multi-network vehicle routers. Retrieved from Sierra Wireless: https://www.sierrawireless.com/products-and-solutions/routers-gateways/mg90/

13. swyMed. *Why swyMed?* Retrieved from swyMed: http://swymed.com/why-swymed-overview/

Chapter 3
Remote Patient Monitoring: Delegation of Responsibility

Elizabeth A. Krupinski and Jaclyn A. Pagliaro

3.1 Introduction

Healthcare is becoming increasingly more technical, not only with respect to the wide array of new devices and tests available to providers and patients, but also the overall healthcare delivery paradigm. The integration of wearable remote monitoring devices and telemedicine is altering the way clinical care is provided and research is conducted. Wearable remote monitoring devices can be deployed to patients and utilized to extend patient data collection outside of conventional clinical encounters [1]. The anticipated impact of remote data collection on patients and health care systems is to increase provider efficacy and efficiency, thereby increasing quality of care [2–4]. This improved quality of life is the result of more reliable and timely methods for collecting, transmitting, and storing personal health data for health care communications. Within this context is the evolution of guidelines for responding to remotely collected and stored data, and reimbursement policies [5, 6] that accommodate remote data management in any reimbursement structures.

Recent research supports the use of RPM for adults with cardiovascular disease demonstrating that consistent blood pressure tracking and communication with healthcare teams improves BP related outcomes. RPM lowers both systolic and diastolic blood pressure more than standard in-office BP management. RPM may also promote early detection of atrial fibrillation and improve heart failure volume and weight management.

E. A. Krupinski (✉)
Department of Radiology & Imaging Sciences, Emory University, Atlanta, GA, USA
e-mail: ekrupin@emory.edu

J. A. Pagliaro
Division of Cardiology, Department of Medicine, Massachusetts General Hospital, Boston, MA, USA
e-mail: jaclyn.pagliaro@mgh.harvard.edu

© Springer Nature Switzerland AG 2021
A. B. Bhatt (ed.), *Healthcare Information Technology for Cardiovascular Medicine*, Health Informatics, https://doi.org/10.1007/978-3-030-81030-6_3

Wearable devices now add to the RPM field and are being designed to collect data about various physiological, psychological and environmental parameters at the individual and population level which complement standard digital medical data acquisition. As these devices proliferate, data is constantly accessible by a variety of parties (e.g., patients, providers, hospitals, vendors), regardless of the location of the individual from whom the data is being recorded. An increasing number of devices can acquire, transmit and store data to enhance the relationship between patients and their providers.

The use of ambulatory monitoring devices in the cardiology setting enables long-term, remote data collection for reliable diagnostics and continuous monitoring of cardiac disease [7]. The device field in cardiology is one of the most advanced of all medical specialties in terms of monitoring and intervention. This provides an existing scaffold for the mechanisms and workflow for remote data collection and analysis, as exemplified in electrophysiology, heart failure, cardiac rehabilitation and most recently in cardio-obstetrics. Remote patient monitoring (RPM) is being used in a variety of applications such as remote monitoring of implantable devices [8] and remote electrocardiogram monitoring [9]. Most studies demonstrate that use of RPM is feasible and can be used to assess device and patient status in a reliable and valid manner. Success may depend on factors such as the type of device (manufacturer, model), patient status, type of information acquired, and even the algorithms used to assess the incoming data (impacting false negative and alarm rates). Thus, some caution should always be used when interpreting RPM data and when to base clinical decisions on the data received. It is particularly important to work with the device manufacturers to understand the criteria used in the various data analysis algorithms used to notify users and providers of significant changes in the data and patient status.

Despite the many advancements, there is still much work that needs to be done in terms of research to improve our understanding of actual outcomes and benefits of these tools. It is also critical to determine which patient populations are best suited to benefit from the use of these devices [10]. On the positive side, patients do seem receptive to remote patient monitoring and are generally satisfied with the experience [11, 12].

A key topic that arises when one thinks about all these data is responsibility. When and in what circumstances is it the provider's responsibility to utilize the acquired data? There is currently no strict legal statute, but there are ways to think about data sources that may be helpful.

3.2   Data and Context

As a first step it is useful to distinguish between data acquired strictly within the context of healthcare encounters and data that could be used for research purposes.

3.2.1 Research Context

Until a formally recommended structure exists regarding acquiring, transmitting and storing various personal and medical sources of data, we should always apply the Belmont Report's guiding principles of human research (Table 3.1) to the use of any personal data [13].

3.2.2 Clinical Context

3.2.2.1 Data Solicited by Providers

Data solicited by providers refers to data that patients collect by wearing a device that acquires and transmits data to their healthcare provider to be used for medical decision-making. In this circumstance, the provider "prescribes" a wearable device to acquire the data.

Data security must ensure that the data are protected from unauthorized users during transfer, collection and processing, and that they are safely stored to protect identifiable health data from unwarranted access or disclosure. Since RPM is wireless, there is the inherent risk that data can be intercepted, tracked and possibly used in harmful or illegal ways. However, devices that are FDA-approved undergo fairly rigorous evaluation [14] with respect to security, so these risks are minimized (usually via data encryption and authentication).

The patient and physician must communicate effectively so the patient understands why, how and when the data are collected, transferred and stored and how they will be used in their care and treatment (Table 3.2). Interestingly, although

Table 3.1 Belmont Report's guiding principles of human research

Three guiding principles for protection of human subjects in Behavioral & Biomedical Research	
Respect for persons	The autonomy of people must be respected in terms of allowing them to make choices and providing informed consent.
Beneficence	Researchers must maximize benefits and minimize risks to those involved.
Justice	Benefits and costs associated with participation must be fairly and equally distributed among all potential participants.

Table 3.2 Recommendations for provider solicited data

- Ensure safety of data acquisition
- Identify any limitations associated with validity and reliability of data
- Recognize variations in use of application with various patient populations
- Understand the nature of false alarms
- Know how to incorporate the output data into clinical decision making diagnosis and treatment

patients do have concerns about the technology itself and security issues they are often more concerned about loss of contact with providers and whether out-of-pocket expenses will be incurred [15]. Therefore, it is important that physicians are aware of such concerns and work with patients to address them [16, 17].

3.2.2.2 Data Not Solicited by Providers

Data that patients generate without a formal request from a provider can come from a variety of sources. Consumers use wearable monitoring devices such as Smartwatches or Fitness Trackers with the expectation that they will impact their health status and often share their data as an adjunct to their care. This data derived from remote monitoring devices has been found to provide valuable insight into the patient's overall health to provide comprehensive treatment and care [18, 19]. When a patient brings data from these types of unsolicited data sources to a healthcare encounter (which could be in-person, through a patient portal, email, text, a video encounter, phone or any other mode), the provider has a choice to make. At the same time, it is also becoming apparent that some patients are often willing to acquire various types of health data, including RPM from both provider-approved and off-the-shelf devices (e.g., FitBits [20], and then publicly post that data on social media outlets, complicating the issue even further [19] as most social media companies actually consider any posted data theirs and thus can do with it as they wish. When a patient brings data from these types of unsolicited data sources to a healthcare encounter (which could be in-person, through a patient portal, email, text, a video encounter, phone or any other mode), the provider has a choice to make: should the data be accepted and stored in the electronic health record or other data repository or should the data be declined and thus not stored? Unfortunately, there are few clear-cut guidelines to help with this choice.

Whereas the patient claims responsibility when they choose to acquire and present data to their provider, the clinician's responsibility is less clear. When data was not requested by the clinician, if they decide to accept and store it in the electronic health record they assume a share of the responsibility for the data. This includes its use in medical decision-making and its security (e.g., HIPAA regulations automatically apply). This creates a series of additional responsibilities such as doing the necessary research to understand the device or tool from which the data were acquired, what the limitations of the data acquisition process are, the data validity and reliability, factors that can influence data quality. Without this additional step it becomes difficult sometimes to responsibly incorporate the data into care.

If the provider chooses not to accept the data, at first glance it seems that they avoid responsibility. There are several mechanisms by which the provider may need to address the data, however:

1. If the patient provides the data to another provider who uses it to change the course of treatment this may reflect on the original clinician who decided not to accept the data.

2. If a clinician later decides to use the data, there is little published guidance as to what their responsibility is for previously stored data.
3. If there are abnormal values, there is no clear legal precedence regarding the clinician's accountability. The next phase of telemedicine and utilization of patient derived data is to offer clinician's guidance with these emerging decisions.

3.3 Wearable Devices and Remote Patient Monitoring in Cardiology

Cardiology is remarkably data driven and most guidelines have algorithms to provide comprehensive patient care. The ability to integrate additional tracking mechanisms into existing workflows has been successful in several healthcare systems. The value of digital health and telemedicine can be best described (Table 3.3) as addressing the trifecta of preventative care, chronic disease management and early detection.

3.4 Patient Driven Tools

One of the fastest growing areas of medical technologies is the commercial availability of health monitoring tools. Activity trackers, Bluetooth enabled BP and HR monitors, mobile ECG, and many other devices have flooded the marketplace. Fitting these tools into a digital heart center introduces unique complexities, as questions of data fidelity, false positive and false negative rates, and helping patients distinguish between data and information all play a much larger role in these technologies than other parts of a technology forward cardiology practice. In addition to the question of what problem does this technology solve, for these technologies, we must also ask the question: what harm comes from inaccurate information?

Table 3.3 Key areas where digital health and telemedicine can address preventative care, chronic disease management and early detection

Prevention	– Wearable devices and telemedicine can improve healthcare access to patients who experience barriers to care
Chronic disease management	– Wearables allow clinicians to continuously manage large patient populations at a distance rather than fewer patients with episodic in-person care alone – Patients with chronic diseases who use wearables and telemedicine also benefit from decreased stress, saved time and finances, while also remaining active members in their local community
Early detection	– Digital health allows early detection of decompensation leading to rapid and targeted intervention – Algorithms can be applied to the collected data to provide remote clinical care such as medication titrations

3.5   What Harm Comes from Inaccurate Information?

If a patient has purchased a health monitoring device on their own, the patient has already signaled that they get some value from the device. So while it's still important to figure out what problem the device solves for the clinical team, it is much more important to figure out how the information on the device (especially if it's inaccurate) could bring harm to the patient.

One of the best examples of such a technology is the new Apple Watch. The apple watch has two features of interest: one is a calorie/activity tracker, that measures activity in a day in "calories burned" and the other is the ECG monitor, which can offer a single lead ECG tracing. For an activity monitor, the accuracy is likely not that important. When the device says the patient burns 500 calories, if the "true" calorie consumption is 300 or 700 calories, it is unlikely to harm the patient. In fact, if it is relatively precise (consistent day to day) and motivates a patient toward more activity, the accuracy of the activity count is largely irrelevant. Incorporating such a tool in a virtual cardiac rehab program, for example, would confer minimal risk for the patient.

> **Case study example:** Thomson et al. examined the Fitbit Charge HR 2 (Fitbit) and Apple Watch devices to assess hea   every vigorous intensities based on ECG-measured HR. Apple Watch showed lower relative error rates (2.4–5. 1%) compared to Fitbit (3.9–13.5%) for all intensities. The strongest relationship for both devices with ECG-measured HR was for very light PA and strength of the relationship declined as exercise intensity increased for both devices. *Thomson EA. Nuss K, Comstock A, Reinwald S, Blake S, Pimentel RE, Tracy BL, Li K. Heart rate measures from the Apple Watch, Fitbit Charge HR2, and electrocardiogram across different exercise intensities. J Sports Sciences 2019; 37:1411-1419*

On the other hand, the ECG tool has a different risk equation. One diagnosis the ECG monitor on the apple watch hopes to make is atrial fibrillation [21]. Here, a false positive diagnosis could result in inappropriate anticoagulant therapy with the associated bleeding risk without potential for benefit. On the other hand, a false negative result could incorrectly reassure us that the patient doesn't have atrial fibrillation, resulting in inadequately withholding anticoagulation therapy. In one estimation, for every 1 patient correctly diagnosed with atrial fibrillation, 19 people potentially would be inappropriately placed on anticoagulation. In this case, the watch could be used as a screening tool, but care should be used in making treatment decisions based on the data.

Since the patient has purchased the device, it has solved at least one problem for them (patient comfort). Still, it's important that the clinical team determine what (if any) problems the device helps them solve. A clear understanding of what we hope to get from a new device and how we communicate that to patients (Table 3.4) helps

Table 3.4 Ambulatory device capabilities and how we communicate that to patients

Ambulatory monitoring capabilities	Considerations for patient communication
Vital sign data sources – Heart rate – Respiratory rate – Temperature – Oxygen saturation – Blood pressure Wearable data streams – ECG – Sleep assessment – Physical activity	Heart rate variability exists, normal ranges should be reviewed with patients FDA approved blood pressure monitors are largely accurate, but checking calibration in the office is useful Oxygen saturation meters can be inaccurate with improper placement At home single lead ECG will not mirror an in-office 12-lead in its entirety for diagnosis. Single lead home ECG or HR monitor devices may have false positives for arrhythmia and follow up with formal ECG or monitoring is recommended before treatment

maximize the benefit for the patient, but also reduces their frustration, as the clinical team can offer up front guidance on what the device can and cannot do.

3.6   Guidance for RPM Workflow Development and Implementation

Cardiology practices should establish an infrastructure for receipt, analysis and clinical application of any form of "remote monitoring". Practices can create an effective and safe mechanism for the use of remote monitoring and wearable device data.

1. All data (whether or not it was requested by the provider) should be subject to the same security and privacy requirements of any patient health information (PHI). This includes hard copies on site or cloud-based data.
2. Organizations should have in place policies and protocols governing the use of any and all types of remote patient monitoring data. The policy should include how and if unsolicited patient generated data will or could be used and what criteria should be used in the decision to accept or not.
3. If providers are going to recommend certain devices or tools be used by patients, they should have a formal program in place that manages the schedule and timing of data collection by the patient, transfer, storage, retrieval, analysis, and feed back to the patient.
4. Providers should not be responsible for training patients on the actual use of devices that they do not recommend.
5. When a technology or device is prescribed, patients should have a responsibility to submit requested data and the provider(s) should take appropriate action when the patient is non-compliant or is unable to participate appropriately.
6. Protocols should be in place regarding alerts generated from remote monitoring devices (especially when artificial intelligence and related decision support tools are used) [22–25]—when to respond to them, who should respond, how the patient should be contacted and what follow-up measures should be in place.

7. Policies should also be in place for all data sources regarding how long the data should be stored.

Some resources are available to providers such as the American Medical Association's "Digital Health Implementation Playbook" that provides a very nice summary of RPM and other digital tools available and how to integrate them into patient care [26].

Cardiac specific workflow for RPM, which incorporates patient solicited data mandates a clear approach to appropriately protect patient data.

First, we must define what data points are clinically relevant and how it will be identified, collected and communicated to the appropriate care team member. Next, organize remote patient monitoring data into existing practice workflows. Finally, do not create new workflows and additional clinical and administrative burden.

For successful implementation (Fig. 3.1), engaging the staff is essential to a successful transformation to a digital RPM inclusive practice. Staff (clinical and administrative) training should include knowledge on how to explain the device role in management, order, deliver and engage with the device from a patient perspective, help troubleshoot and have access to the device manufacturers helpline. Practices will also need to be able to schedule device checks and data downloads, oversee data acquisition, be familiar with patient information materials and most importantly, know when to contact clinicians.

A successful patient-clinician partnership is the first and most important outcome to achieve during a transition to increased RPM usage in the practice. Patients need to be equal partners in device use, understand clinical endpoints that are being measured and be facile with methods of communication with the clinical team. Although some recommend patient selection for compliance and technological proficiency, the goal of expanding care to the individual patient is to improve access, therefore we must meet patients and help overcome their barriers. Addressing social determinants of health is a foundational part of the patient engagement strategy.

Once a successful partnership is achieved and demonstrated, outcomes then include a range of clinical, experiential and business outcomes (Table 3.5).

The National Institute for Standards and Technology [27] is also addressing some RPM issues and has posted a request for "technology vendors to participate in the development of an example solution for securing the telehealth remote

Structure	Process	Outcomes
For successful RPM, data points and workflow must be well-defined	All members of the practice, administrative and clinical, will require training and ongoing technical and clinical support for successful implementation of RPM	Patient and physician satisfaction, use of the RPM system, increased access and achievement of clinical endpoints can be sequentially evaluated as an RPM program is established.

Fig. 3.1 Steps for successful implementation of RPM use

Table 3.5 Clinical, experiential and business outcomes for successful RPM implementation

Clinical outcomes	• Blood pressure monitoring
	• HF exacerbation management
	• Admission and readmission Reduction
	• GDMT achievement regardless of cardiac diagnosis
	• Compliance with medications
	• Improved clinical markers of disease
	• Less progression of disease
Experiential outcomes	• Patient, staff and provider satisfaction
	• Accessing healthcare appointments
	• Successful engagement with interpreter services
	• Coordinated multidisciplinary visits patient engagement with technology
Business outcomes	• Decreased cancellations and no shows
	• Increased clinical productivity
	• Fewer hospitalizations and ED utilization
	Telemedicine utilization
	Reimbursement

patient monitoring ecosystem" to create a Cybersecurity Practice Guide. The European Commission [28] is also developing frameworks for mHealth guidance that includes RPM.

RPM implementation requires several steps for success. Adequately supporting the technology, workflow and staffing for an RPM program is essential for sustainability. Unlike the use of synchronous telemedicine for expanding access and improving outcomes by reaching more patients, the use of RPM requires well-selected populations with effective patient-clinician communication and adequate staff resourcing to demonstrate clinical efficacy and improve outcomes.

Similar to clinical trials, establishing an RPM program requires inclusion and exclusion criteria for patient enrollment, as well as the equivalent of shared decision making, wherein patients understand the goal of RPM, and the importance of their active role to enable success. The initial onboarding for all telemedicine modalities, whether synchronous video, text-based interactions, or RPM including wearable data needs to be a personal one-on-one thorough explanation at the initiation of the program, with continued opportunity for contacting the team for troubleshooting on demand. Even one poor interaction with telemedicine risks creating an aversion to its use. However the stakes are higher with RPM, in that one poor interaction may result in less than optimal care.

Key Steps in Implementation of RPM (Table 3.6):

- Administrative staff, leadership and clinical staff must all be involved in design review prior to implementation
- Patients should understand the goal of RPM for their healthcare and their role in a successful model of care
- Real-time, at the elbow help for administrative, workflow and technical assistance must be in place not only at implementation but in some form for the duration of chronic disease management using RPM.

Table 3.6 Key common sense steps in implementation of RPM

Common-sense steps to implemention an RPM wearable device program:
- Establish program structure, process and outcomes to be measured
- Center the program around specific patient populations
- Document data acquisition and data use in the clinical decision-making process
- Guarantee security and privacy
- Support data entry by patients, providers and staff where applicable
- Provide links to patient records to facilitate full data ineqration
- Incorporate clinical guidelines in establishing criteria for responding to alarms based on the data (for example, agree upon published acceptable false positive and false negative rates)
- Document procedures for data alarms including who is screening, in what time frame is a response needed, what to do when a patient does not respond, how to document the response
- Determine who is responsible for the data (acquiring, transmitting, storing) and engage your legal tream regarding clinical responsibility and interaction with industry
- Determine how long RPM data should be collected and stored (and how much of it)

3.7 Conclusions

There is no doubt that RPM techniques and wearable devices will continue to be developed and implemented by providers and patients in a wide variety of clinical applications, including cardiology [29]. Although the potential for improving patient outcomes with these devices is high, the evidence on outcomes to date is still inconclusive in many respects [30, 31]. More large-scale studies (e.g., [32]) are required to better assess the impact of RPM and wearables devices in broader, more heterogeneous groups of patients with a variety of cardiovascular conditions and degrees of severity. As we proceed down this path as a healthcare community that includes not only providers but also patients and their caregivers, we need to continue to develop and refine our perspectives and guidance surrounding the ethical, sage and effective use of virtual data no matter what its source. Remote patient data ownership must be considered, but it should not represent a barrier or hindrance in its use as a tool to improve the efficacy and efficiency of clinical decision making and the care and treatment of patients.

References

1. DeVore AD, Wosik J, Hernandez AF. The future of wearables in heart failure patients. JACC Heart Fail. 2019;7(11):922–32.
2. Liao Y, Thompson P, Peterson S, Mandrola J, Shaalan M. The future of wearable technologies and remote monitoring in health care. Am Soc Clin Oncol Educ Book. 2019:115–21.
3. Malasinghe L, Ramzan N, Dahal K. Remote patient monitoring: a comprehensive review. J Ambient Intell Humaniz Comput. 2019;10:57–76.
4. Queiros A, Alvarelhao J, Cerqueira M, Silva AG, Santos M, Rocha NP. Remote care technology: a systematic review of reviews and meta-analyses. Technologies. 2018;6:22.

5. Berridge C. Medicaid becomes the first third-party payer to cover passive remote monitoring for home care: policy analysis. J Med Internet Res. 2018;20:e66.
6. Centers for Medicare & Medicaid Services (CMS). 2019 Physician Fee Schedule and Quality Payment Program. 2018. https://www.cms.gov/newsroom/fact-sheets/finalized-policy-payment-and-quality-provisions-changes-medicare-physician-fee-schedule-calendar. Accessed 13 Dec 2019.
7. Sana F, Isselbacher EM, Singh JP, Heist EK, Pathik B, Armoundas AA. Wearable devices for ambulatory cardiac monitoring: JACC state-of-the-art review. J Am Coll Cardiol. 2020;75(13):1582–92.
8. Cheung CC, Deyell MW. Remote monitoring of cardiac implantable electronic devices. Can J Cardiol. 2018;34:941–4.
9. Li J, Yang P, Fu D, Ye X, Zhang L, Chen G, Yang Y, Luo H, Chen L, Shao M, Li C, Liu Y, Zhou Y, Jiang H, Li X. Effects of home-based cardiac exercise rehabilitation with remote electrocardiogram monitoring in patients with chronic heart failure: a study protocol for a randomized controlled trial. BMJ Open. 2019;9:e023923.
10. Dickinson MG, Allen LA, Albert NA, DiSalvo T, Ewald GA, Vest AR, Whellan DJ, Zile MR, Givertz MM. Remote monitoring of patients with heart failure: a white paper from the Heart Failure Society of America Scientific Statements Committee. J Card Fail. 2018;24:682–94.
11. Artico J, Zecchin M, Zorzin Fantasia A, Skerl G, Ortis B, Franco S, Albani S, Barbati G, Cristalli J, Cannata A, Sinagra G. Long-term patient satisfaction with implanted device remote monitoring: a comparison among different systems. J Cardiovasc Med. 2019;20:542–50.
12. Catalan-Matamoros D, Lopez-Villegas A, Tore-Lappegard K, Lopez-Liria R. Patients' experiences of remote communication after pacemaker implant: the NORDLAND study. PLoS One. 2019;14:e0219584.
13. National Commission for the Protection of Human Subjects of Biomedical and Behavioral Research. The Belmont Report: ethical principles and guidelines for the protection of human subjects of research. Bethesda, MD: US Government Printing Office; 1978.
14. United States Food & Drug Administration. Device software functions including mobile medical applications. https://www.fda.gov/medical-devices/digital-health/device-software-functions-including-mobile-medical-applications. Accessed 13 Dec 2019.
15. Walker RC, Tong A, Howard K, Palmer SC. Patient expectations and experiences of remote monitoring for chronic diseases: systematic review and thematic synthesis of qualitative studies. Int J Med Inform. 2019;124:78–85.
16. Maher NA, Senders JT, Hulsbergen AFC, Lamba N, Parker M, Onella JP, Bredenoord AL, Smith TR, Broekman MLD. Passive data collection and use in healthcare: A systematic review of ethical issues. Int J Med Inform. 2019;129:242–7.
17. Mittelstadt B. Ethics of the health-related internet of things: a narrative review. Ethics Inf Technol. 2017;19:157–75.
18. Bierman AS. Functional status: the sixth vital sign. J Gen Intern Med. 2001;1611:785–6.
19. Petersen C, DeMuro P. Legal and regulatory considerations associated with use of patient-generated health data from social media and mobile health (mHealth) devices. Appl Clin Inform. 2015;6:16–26.
20. Thomson EA, Nuss K, Comstock A, Reinwald S, Blake S, Pimentel RE, Tracy BL, Li K. Heart rate measures from the apple watch, Fitbit charge HR 2, and electrocardiogram across different exercise intensities. J Sports Sci. 2019;37(12):1411–9.
21. Turakhia MP, Desai M, Hedlin H, Rajmane A, Talati N, Ferris T, Desai S, Nag D, Patel M, Kowey P, Rumsfeld JS, Russo AM, Hills MT, Granger CB, Mahaffey KW, Perez MV. Rationale and design of a large-scale, app-based study to identify cardiac arrhythmias using a smartwatch: the Apple Heart Study. Am Heart J. 2019;207:66–75.
22. Balthazar P, Harri P, Prater A, Safdar NM. Protecting your patients' interests in the era of big data, artificial intelligence, and predictive analytics. J Am Coll Radiol. 2018;15:580–6.

23. Faden RR, Kass NE, Goodman SN, Pronovost P, Tunis S, Beauchamp TL. An ethics framework for a learning health care system: a departure from traditional research ethics and clinical ethics. Hastings Cent Rep. 2013:S16–27.
24. Geis JR, Brady AP, Wu CC, Spencer J, Ranschaert E, Jaremko JL, Langer SG, Kitts AB, Birch J, Shields WF, van den Hoven van Genderen R, Kotter E, Jochoya JW, Cook TS, Morgan MB, Tang A, Safdar NM, Kohli M. Ethics of artificial intelligence in radiology: summary of the Joint European and North American Multisociety Statement. Radiology. 2019;293:436–40.
25. Wang L, Alexander CA. Big data analytics in biometrics and healthcare. J Comput Sci Appl. 2018;6:48–55.
26. American Medical Association. Digital implementation playbook. 2018. https://www.ama-assn.org/amaone/ama-digital-health-implementation-playbook. Accessed 25 Dec 2019.
27. National Institute for Standards and Technology. Securing the telehealth remote patient monitoring ecosystem. https://www.nccoe.nist.gov/sites/default/files/library/project-descriptions/hit-th-project-description-final.pdf. Accessed 25 Dec 2019.
28. European Commission. Privacy code of conduct on mobile health apps. https://ec.europa.eu/digital-single-market/en/privacy-code-conduct-mobile-health-apps. Accessed 25 Dec 2019.
29. American Heart Association. Using remote patient monitoring technologies for better cardiovascular disease outcomes guidance. 2019. https://www.heart.org/-/media/files/about-us/policy-research/policy-positions/clinical-care/remote-patient-monitoring-guidance-2019.pdf?la=en&hash=A98793D5A04AB9940424B8FB91D2E8D5A5B6BEB. Accessed 25 Dec 2019.
30. Brahmbhatt DH, Cowie MR. Remote management of heart failure: an overview of telemonitoring technologies. Card Fail Rev. 2019;5:86–92.
31. Noah B, Keller MS, Mosadeghi S, Stein L, Johl S, Delshad S, Tashjian VC, Lew D, Kwan JT, Jusufagic A, Spiegel BMR. Impact of remote patient monitoring on clinical outcomes: an updated meta-analysis of randomized controlled trials. NPJ Digit Med. 2018;1:20172.
32. Shufelt C, Dzubur E, Joung S, Fuller G, Mouapi KN, Van Den Broek I, Lopez M, Dhawan S, Arnold CW, Speier W, Mastali M, Fu Q, Van Eyk JE, Spiegel B, Merz CNB. A protocol integrating remote patient monitoring patient reported outcomes and cardiovascular biomarkers. Digital Med. 2019;2:84.

Chapter 4
Building the Digital Heart Center

Ameya Kulkarni

4.1 Introduction

Norman Rockwell did not need technology to capture the soul of doctoring in his iconic painting, "Doctor and the Doll." The painting, which depicts a doctor using his stethoscope to listen to the doll of a frightened young patient, reveals the best of what it means to be a physician—the chance to heal, but also the chance to be present during a patient's most vulnerable moments. There is sometimes a fear that technology, and in particular remote care technology, diminishes this gift our patients give to us. However at its best, technology offers the chance for deeper connections that cross the bounds of time and space. Virtual care can allow us to take care of even our sickest patients from their homes with minimal interruption to their daily lives.

Even for those that see this opportunity in telemedicine, the gap between a belief that virtual care will be helpful and the actual implementation of technologies to support that cause can feel very wide. Narrowing the gap requires a process to define the problems to be solved, navigate the myriad of new technologies, understand how these technologies can help our patients, and create systems to evaluate whether they actually did. Connecting these pillars with the core values of your practice are critical to building a successful and effective digital heart center.

A. Kulkarni (✉)
Mid-Atlantic Permanente Medical Group, Rockville, MD, USA
e-mail: amey.r.kulkarni@kp.org

© Springer Nature Switzerland AG 2021   51
A. B. Bhatt (ed.), *Healthcare Information Technology for Cardiovascular Medicine*, Health Informatics, https://doi.org/10.1007/978-3-030-81030-6_4

Table 4.1 Four questions for stakeholders

Defining question	Crowd-sourced answers	Influence on platform development
What do we do now that makes our work easier?	Use of telephone and secure messages to communicate with patients	When developing a digital platform, having an existing modality of patient communication, will negate the need to build one directly into the application
What are "the pebbles in our shoes" (the things that make our job harder)?	Prior authorization, (CV staff meeting)	
What do we wish we didn't need to do in this workflow?	Manually collect and review vital signs	The platform has to not only collect data (ie, HR, BP, weight) but also present it in a way that reduced the burden of sifting through them
What are the core issues in our workflow that negatively affect the patient experience?	Long patient wait times and limited access to timely data for an initial visit.	Virtual care schedules should be designed to improve access and align with image sharing programs. This allows clinical teams to have timely and clinically meaningful conversations.

4.2 Defining the Problem

Cardiologists love technology. Our interest in quickly adapting new tools in our armament has allowed us to innovate care at a rate unparalleled in other fields. While this is often an asset in the care of our patients, when it comes to virtual care technologies, this can turn into a "shiny object trap." The risk of trying new tools without understanding how they help our core practice or advance our core values results in expensive solutions to small or non-existent problems and eventually a graveyard of discarded shiny objects.

Defending against this trap requires deliberation. It starts with a decidedly non-technical conversation. Prior to incorporating new technologies into our practice, we take a moment to define *the problem we hope to solve* with the technology. This helps identify whether a potential technology will be useful to us, but also helps us guard against the shiny object trap.

Clearly establishing the problem to be solved is challenging. It requires input from people who understand the core values of the practice but also people who live the status quo.

4.3 Understanding the Technology

Once the problem(s) have been defined, the next step is identifying the technologies best suited to address identified needs. Technology is constantly evolving, but most tools for virtual care fit into one of three categories: communication, data collection, and patient initiated.

4.3.1   Data Collection Tools

The modern heart center requires more than discussions with patients. Home measurement of blood pressure and heart rate for patients with hypertension and coronary disease, weight and activity for heart failure patients, and even food journals for patients in virtual cardiac rehab programs are valuable adjuncts to routine care that can significantly improve the way we take care of cardiac patients. But collecting this data in a way that protects patient privacy and presenting it in a way that is useful to clinicians can take time, money, and some understanding of the technical and legal framework surrounding remote monitoring technology.

At its simplest iteration though, minimal work is required. For example, a blood pressure collection system that asks the patient to measure their own BPs on a home machine and relay the data to the clinical care team via telephone or email offers a simple, inexpensive solution. If the problem to be solved is one of simplified and inexpensive data collection on a small scale, this solution will be adequate.

As the scale or complexity of such a project increases, the work of verifying adherence to self-reporting and tracking becomes exponentially more difficult [1]. For these situations, more complex solutions are required. For example, when building a large remote monitoring program for patients across an enterprise with uncontrolled hypertension, there are three key values (Mid Atlantic Permanente Medical Group) that we considered mission critical:

1. The data collected has to be collected, transmitted and reported in a way that protects the patient's privacy from end to end.
2. The process of signing up, transmitting data and dis-enrolling from the program should be easy for the patient and clinician.
3. Given the volume of data that would come to clinician dashboards, the reporting workbench had to be easy to navigate and contain "passive alerts" – which meant the system would signal the clinician when a reading was abnormal or when the patient was non-adherent to measurements, so that clinicians would not have to continually check dashboards for hundreds or thousands of people.

Defining the problem ahead of the technology allows prioritization of what is needed for the minimum viable product (MVP) [2] and sets expectations for clinical teams. Once a roadmap is outlined, clinicians are willing to wait for iterative versions improving workflow (See example, Fig. 4.1).

Of course, between a manual collection of blood pressure readings and a complex automated and integrated BP monitoring system are hundreds of technical solutions with varying degrees of complexity. Starting with the problems and following with the technology offers the chance to fit the solution for the right situation.

Sample Clinical Workflow for Clinical Telemedicine Visits

This diagram demonstrates a sample clinical algorithm to enable delivery of virtual medical care
and highlights opportunities to streamline workflows administratively to unburden physicians.

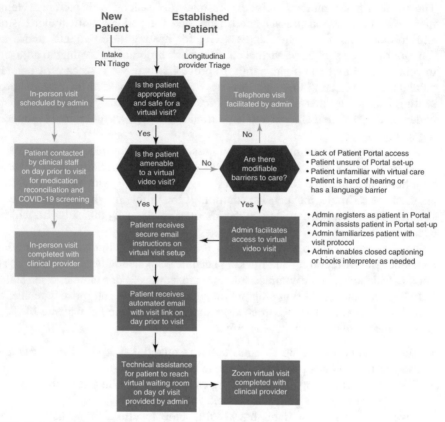

Source: Massachusetts General Hospial, Division of Cardiology

Fig. 4.1 Sample clinical workflow for clinical telemedicine visits

4.4 Implementation

Building a strategic framework and defining the technologies set the theoretical
groundwork for a digital heart center. The next phase, implementation, requires
careful attention to regulatory considerations, clear definitions of what success and
failure is, a willingness to iterate solutions as new information comes about, and
an accounting for the unique personality mix among the clinicians in your practice.

4.4.1 Regulatory Considerations

The most challenging aspect of offering virtual care is navigating the regulatory framework. At the local, state, and federal level, policies governing privacy, delivery of medical care, and handling of collected data are complicated and in the COVID-19 era, rapidly changing. The reality is that it is nearly impossible for clinicians to navigate these complexities. You will need help from institutional partners who are experts in technology risk, medical law, and compliance. In our experience, involving these experts early in the discussion, even as we are outlining the problem, helps bound our solution in what is possible, making the process significantly more efficient. These partners also help us favor simplicity, which means digital health tools can be evaluated without significant initial investment.

4.4.2 Monitoring and Evaluation

A common trap in the early phases of building a digital health program is to start trying a technology without deciding what defines a successful tool, and what warrants abandonment of the idea. To combat this instinct, we begin implementation with the following questions:

1. How do we know if this new tool is a success?
2. How do we know if this new tool is a failure?
3. What is our criteria to expand?
4. What is our criteria to abandon?

A critical step in answering these questions is to be as specific as possible. It is also important to be realistic. With new technologies, and in particular remote monitoring devices, there is a deep belief that technology can result in clinical improvement. Unfortunately, the data has not borne that out [3–5]. Empirically this makes sense, as remote monitoring tools don't offer new information, but rather make that information easier to obtain. So defining success by other targets (such as increasing healthy days at home or improving patient satisfaction) may be more meaningful goals for the technology.

As important as defining success is defining failure. Once deep into a pilot project, there is a natural inclination to "make it work," often by adding financial or other investments. By defining a priori when the costs of the project or the results favor abandonment, it creates an honest arbiter of failure, and in the long run reduces the costs of those failures.

4.4.3   Iterations

Technology companies often define the first version of any product as the minimum viable product (MVP). This concept gives permission for a new idea to not be perfect at first attempt, but also helps identify what needs to be perfect first, before other aspects of the product can be worked on. In designing digital health tools, a similar framework is necessary. Often the first version of a product will only solve the basic technical and regulatory challenges. Walking through the markers of success and the minimum requirements for each iteration are important, but most important is to acknowledge that there will be multiple iterations before a fully functioning technologic solution works as intended.

4.4.4   Gaining Support for Widespread Adoption

Even the best of ideas need to be used by clinicians to be successful. Like technology adoption in any realm, digital health tools have an adoption curve. Innovators and Early adopters are willing to try new technology and will be willing to engage and re-engage, even when a tool is not functioning perfectly. Mainstream users (early and late majority) need a polished product but will tolerate some challenges. Late adopters require a nearly seamless experience and a well established workflow (Fig. 4.2). Part of any implementation strategy should include identification of which clinicians fit each of these categories for the technology being deployed. Since comfort with new tools is not monolithic—someone may be very comfortable with video visit technology but may not feel as comfortable with a remote monitoring platform—where clinicians fall on the adoption curve should be assessed with every roll out. Once the groups have been identified, roll out should follow the curve, with early adopters getting their first chance at trying the new solution and offering feedback on what doesn't work. Feedback from late adopters will be useful as well, because when the solution takes a life of its own, the feedback from late adopters will help identify where the potential gaps lie.

Central figure: Key steps in Building a Digital heart center

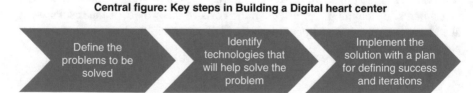

Fig. 4.2 Key steps in building a Digital Hearth Center

4.5 Summary

Conversations on building a digital heart center often focus on the technology to be deployed. It is the fidelity of the ECG tracing on an Apple Watch, or the computing power of machine learning that dominates the discussion. But when a more systematic approach is applied, starting with identification of the problems to be solved, bolstered by careful selection of technology, and executed through an implementation plan that accounts for success measures and the clinicians responsible for using the technology, something bigger happens. The technology becomes a vehicle to solve the problems that all of us face in busy modern cardiology practices—how to diagnose and treat disease as quickly and efficiently as possible, how to streamline data collection so that treatment plans can focus on the patient needs, and most importantly, how to leverage modern tools to build deep and meaningful connections with our patients. At its best, the digital heart center gives us a chance to repaint Rockwell's doctor on a modern canvas.

Case Studies
In the following case studies, apply the framework from this chapter to design a technology based solution to problems commonly seen in modern cardiology practices. The discussion accompanying the case study is not meant to reflect a "correct" answer as there are many possible and viable approaches.

Case 1: Your cardiology practice has noted a poor adherence rate to a traditional hospital based post myocardial infarction cardiac rehab program, with completion rates at 7%. Your team decides to design a virtual home based cardiac rehab program based in your office.

Question 1: What core problem do you hope to solve in this program?
Question 2: What technologies are required to accomplish your goal?
Question 3: How will you know you are successful?
Question 4: Design a program that would work in your practice.

Discussion: In this case, the core issue was adherence to the program. While patients were being referred at a high rate and were attending their first sessions with consistency, by week 6 of the hospital based program, the rigors of needing to go to the hospital three times a week made adherence difficult. When we took stock of what worked well already and where the pain points were, we discovered that patients liked the guidance with exercise and regular contact with their rehab team, but felt that the rehab program was disconnected from the office practice and most importantly, they wished for an exercise program they could do at home. So the core problem to solve was to design a rehab program that allowed patients to safely exercise at home.

Interestingly, the technology to achieve such a goal was minimal. A twelve week program with an initial discussion of an exercise plan (after a stress test to establish baseline exertional tolerance) and regular check ins via phone solved the problem. Initially we discussed including an app based rehab program that collected activity and BP/weight data, but understanding that while interesting, that technology did not solve our core problem meant that we held off. The reduced technical lift meant that we were able to quickly deploy and expand a virtual home based cardiac rehab program with minimal financial investment.

Defining success in this case stemmed from the core problem, which was completion adherence. We knew if we had a program with a higher rate of completion than 7%, we would have a successful program. Amazingly, after 1 year, our completion percentage was >70%.

One lesson for me in the design of our virtual cardiac rehab program was that technology should fit the core solution. In this case, the most appropriate initial tool was a telephone, despite the availability of shinier objects! Recognizing this early meant more rapid deployment at a significantly lower cost.

Case 2: The electrophysiologist in your practice has been wondering about a new way to consult on patients who need primary prevention devices. He is interested in minimizing the amount they need to travel to see him, and because he notes the physical exam doesn't add much to a consultation to discuss device placement, he has been wondering about virtual methods of consultation. However, he says that the device battery itself is an important and useful part of the consent discussion, and so is concerned about the use of virtual consults.

Question 1: What is the core problem?
Question 2: What are the potential communication tools that can be used to
                 solve the problem at hand? Which one will work the best?

Discussion: In this circumstance, understanding more detail about the core problem helped elucidate the right solution. In asking the electrophysiologist what about the device was useful, he said that it was seeing the device that gave the most information. Understanding the dimensions of the battery offered patients who were anxious about having the implant some comfort. Evaluating virtual communication tools through this lens made the answer obvious—while a secure message with a picture would solve the visual problem, it wouldn't allow for a conversation/informed consent. A telephone call would lose the visual portion, so a video consult was the optimal solution. By doing video consultations for new devices, patients could comfortably understand the risks of their upcoming procedure without being burdened with a drive to the office.

Case 3: Your traditional cardiology practice has been disrupted by a global pandemic of a highly infectious disease. You are particularly concerned about patients presenting to hospital emergency rooms with rapid atrial fibrillation, as these patients are most vulnerable to the infectious disease. Your organization is supportive in helping you build a home based hospital program for patients with rapid atrial fibrillation but has asked you to design a solution.

Question 1: What are the core problem(s) to be solved?
Question 2: What technologies will be required to build such a program? What other resources will be needed?
Question 3: How will you measure success?

Discussion: A highly relevant problem in 2020. The answers to these questions will vary by practice and by population, but for our practice, the core problem was safely managing patients with rapid atrial fibrillation outside the hospital. What this meant for us was the ability to (1) Be sure the patient was safe to be home (2) monitor heart rate periodically (3) Administer oral medications intermittently and (4) Connect with the patients virtually 1–2 times per day as needed. These four considerations structured the problems to be solved and thus the solution.

To begin with, we needed to define who would be safe to go home. Because rapid atrial fibrillation is a condition of symptoms in most cases (and not a life threatening arrhythmia), we could use entry criteria for a home based hospital program to set safety guardrails. Patients with hemodynamic instability or evidence of heart failure, for example, would not be candidates for a home based program. Delving deeper into our heart rate monitoring requirements, we realized that medication titration really only required a measurement of pulse and BP—parameters that a patient could be taught to do in the ED prior to discharge. Doses of oral medications could be sent home with the patient for titration under the guidance of a physician and virtual connections could be established using our existing virtual tools (telephone/video/secure messages).

Definition of success for us was solving the patient's problem without requiring hospitalization.

In this case, having an existing framework to design new solutions meant that we could quickly adapt to a seismic shift in the landscape of care in a safe and measured way.

References

1. Bhandari A, Wagner T. Self-reported utilization of health care services: improving measurement and accuracy. Med Care Res Rev. 2006;63(2):217–35. https://doi.org/10.1177/1077558705285298.
2. https://healthcare.mckinsey.com/why-evolving-healthcare-services-and-technology-market-matters

3. Perez MV, Mahaffey KW, Hedlin H, et al. Large-scale assessment of a smartwatch to identify atrial fibrillation. N Engl J Med. 2019;381:1909–17.
4. https://twitter.com/venkmurthy/status/1042142046402891776?s=20
5. Chaudhry SI, Mattera JA, Curtis JP, et al. Telemonitoring in patients with heart failure [published correction appears in N Engl J Med. 2011 Feb 3;364(5):490] [published correction appears in N Engl J Med. 2013 Nov 7;369(19):1869]. N Engl J Med. 2010;363(24):2301–9. https://doi.org/10.1056/NEJMoa1010029.

Chapter 5
Financial Value for Cardiovascular Telemedicine

Andrew Watson and Ritu Thamman

Telemedicine has been present in healthcare for over 20 years, and initially it solved fundamental challenges and focused on the technical aspects that enabled it. Starting with the digital era revolution in the United States, the time between 2007 and 2015 saw a technological transformation. This digital transformation enabled hospitals, doctors, patients, and all the types of telemedicine and created a new horizon for virtual clinical delivery. This new view of telemedicine began to surface our understanding of its financial value.

Healthcare, at its most fundamental level, is dedicated to providing healthcare for patients, and it is based on business models. Therefore, telemedicine is providing care for sick patients and also providing well care, but it has to follow a sound financial model. The rise of the technical capabilities of telemedicine has enabled financial experts to begin to understand the long-term and more holistic model that incorporates telemedicine into the business of healthcare. Telemedicine continues to evolve, primarily through remote patient monitoring, and the outcomes are growing in terms of volume and a level of sophistication. Therefore we have reached a crucial point in telemedicine where virtual activity must be based on financial models with a sound economic underpinning.

All the major cardiovascular diagnoses can be impacted by telemedicine: CHF, AFib, CAD/STEMI, and HTN. The COVID era of March through May of 2020 forced healthcare almost entirely to be delivered through telemedicine. There were services such as surgery or face-to-face emergency care, which followed the traditional in-person methodologies. Still, in essence, the rest of the delivery system went virtual in an emergent fashion. This gave us a unique perspective on

A. Watson
Department of Surgery, University of Pittsburgh Medical Center, Pittsburgh, PA, USA
e-mail: watsar@upmc.edu

R. Thamman (✉)
Department of Medicine, University of Pittsburgh School of Medicine, Pittsburgh, PA, USA

© Springer Nature Switzerland AG 2021   61
A. B. Bhatt (ed.), *Healthcare Information Technology for Cardiovascular Medicine*, Health Informatics, https://doi.org/10.1007/978-3-030-81030-6_5

telemedicine's financial value and accelerated the adoption of telemedicine throughout the United States. As the first wave of COVID slowed in June 2020, the healthcare systems looked to understand the new norm, which is a combination of telemedicine and face-to-face encounters, all of which are based on the financial model behind telemedicine [1]. With cardiovascular medicine for both sick and patients, telemedicine represents a significant opportunity to provide value and, in particular financial benefit.

Financial value falls under the broader rubric of value as a whole, and value is defined as the cost of healthcare combined with the quality healthcare. The cost of healthcare is based on the unit price and the rate of utilization. Therefore, telemedicine's financial value for cardiovascular care can be impacted by changing the unit cost, the rate of utilization, and quality of care metrics, which increase in importance. The quality of care is a critical feedback loop for the financing of healthcare, for both the hospital and payer side. Hospital and payer quality metrics govern the high-level funding of all healthcare. Therefore, when we discuss cardiovascular telemedicine care's financial value, the quality of care is an important consideration. Now that telemedicine is becoming more commonplace and more central throughout healthcare, defining its monetary value is critical not only for how payers, providers and hospitals use it today but also in long-term tactical integration. The year 2020 represents a landmark year for the deployment of telemedicine. Still, behind the scenes, it also represents the defining moment for how we position time telemedicine for financial value moving forward.

Cardiovascular medicine has been at the forefront of innovation to advance patient care during the digital era revolution in the United States. The cardiovascular digital transformation enabled the creation of a new horizon for virtual cardiac care delivery. As infrastructure changed, telemedicine required the development of a financial model to parallel the novel care paradigms. The implementation of telemedicine has the potential to cut healthcare costs by an estimated $7 billion a year in the United States alone [2].

Financial leaders in institutions and practices now must devise a long-term model that incorporates telemedicine into the business of healthcare. During the COVID-19 era of March through May 2020 healthcare was forced to be almost entirely virtual. There were services such as surgery or in-person emergency care, which followed the traditional in-person methodologies however, the rest of the delivery system went virtual in an emergent fashion. This gave us a unique perspective on telemedicine's financial value and accelerated the adoption of telemedicine throughout the United States.

Reducing or containing the cost of healthcare is one of the strongest motivators to fund and adopt virtual care technologies. Telehealth reduces the cost of healthcare and increases efficiency with better management of chronic diseases, shared health professional staffing, reduced travel times, and fewer or shorter hospital stays. Telemedicine's financial value for cardiovascular care can be impacted by changing the unit cost, the rate of utilization, and quality of care metrics. Hospital and payer quality metrics govern how we define monetary value and are critical in establishing how payers, providers and hospitals create a blended and in person care model.

5.1   Defining Financial Value in Telemedicine

Telemedicine has three key facets, which influence integration into clinical cardio-vascular care and financial value. Clinical outcomes, access to care and patient experience are all essential to financial success. The recent history of telecardiology has evolved over the past two decades. From 2000 to 2010, synchronous video visits to live rural clinics, access to care over broadband, remote EKG readings, tele-echocardiography and video consultations were predominant. The payment meth-odologies were often standard contracting fees for subspecialty cardiac care. The system wide downstream value of expanding outreach using these remote clinics was significant and allowed programs to continue, though not necessarily expand, especially as reimbursement rates were limited by rural local designation.

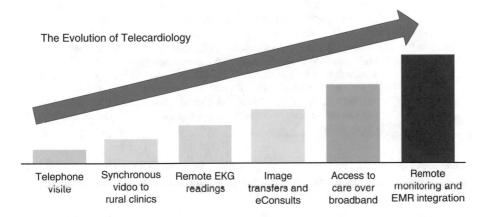

Each of these three areas (asynchronous, live video-based and RPM care) of telemedicine has financial implications for the field of cardiovascular medicine, and each in a very different way (Table 5.1). As these three areas evolve, their integra-tion into the healthcare systems and physician offices will impact the root level finances of healthcare. They may add more capability for encounter and manage-ment billing, they might provide significant value for risk arrangements such as pay for performance, or they could play a significant role for cost avoidance which is a positive in a bundle type setting or a negative for reducing hospital utilization. Therefore, watching the evolution of telemedicine and understanding the basis for its financial value is critical for cardiovascular virtual care evolution.

In the wake of COVID-19, the use of telemedicine grew exponentially causing the value of telemedicine to increase. Catalyzed by necessity and supported by emergent regulatory implementations, many cardiology practices globally transi-tioned to primarily virtual care for some portion of 2020. This has allowed health-care systems to see the potential financial benefit of telemedicine deployment on a large scale. The two most influential factors in creating a positive financial impact using cardiovascular telemedicine are space utilization and clinician top-of-license

Table 5.1 Types of telemedicine tools

Store and Forward Asynchronous Care:	During the early 2000s, methodologies such as teleradiology and store-and-forward technologies became the norm. A similar approach in cardiovascular imaging and electrophysiology monitoring is now utilized for capturing data in remote geographic locations. It reduces workforce redundancy which is appealing to hospitals with low margins who cannot afford to have underutilized physicians at remote sites.
Live Video-based Care:	From 2010 to 2015 this new type of telemedicine evolved based on the maturation of consumer-electronics, cellular technology and smartphones. Although it was initially used in the urgent care setting, this technology has become incorporated into electronic health records (EHRs) and the basis for large telemedicine platform delivery companies such as Teladoc. MD Live and American Well. There are key features developed around the live video visits such as waiting rooms, documentation, and registration that enable large cohorts of patients to be seen by multiple providers akin to a normal busy clinic. During the COVID-19 pandemic, the hospital and doctor financial revenue became almost entirely dependent on this technology.
Remote Patient Monitoring [RPM]:	This is an asynchronous form of telemedicine where data is gathered from a patient at home or a remote location, the data is filtered by a central intake setting such as a call center and is fed into source systems such as EHRs. In comparison to face-to-face visits for data gathering such as BP measurement in a clinic, these systems allow practices to monitor many patients simultaneously, for example allowing rapid iterations of BP medication adjustments leading to shorter time to guideline directed medical therapy and target goals [3].

care. Optimizing these factors has long driven cost savings in outpatient medicine, and the use of virtual care clearly supports decreased space utilization and increased staff engagement [4].

5.2 Financial Impact of Telemedicine Based on Location of Care

Telecardiology care delivery influences the financial impact of the provision of virtual care. There is data supporting the financial impact of both hospital-based and outpatient care models of in-person care and now telemedicine, with each demonstrating unique financial advantages and challenges. The cost of implementation and maintenance of telemedicine systems must be incorporated into the value equation. The use of in hospital telemedicine allows for increased community based care, maximizing the physical use of those locations, while expanding expert clinician reach. The development of efficient telemedicine clinics reduce clinical revenue and increase operational expense, thus adequate design and implementation is critical. The consumer-electronics market has enabled patients to purchase their own phones, wireless plans, computers and broadband plans that minimize the financial outlay for hospitals and outpatient offices for home telemedicine. Much of the expense for patients at home is "free", which is a major benefit for scaling all types of home-based telemedicine for cardiovascular care. Thus the connectivity and integration of telemedicine from the provider side has a real expense, which is partially offset by consumers handing the cost of their endpoints. In low socioeconomic settings, communities and employers may need to partner with hospitals and patients by investing in the technology infrastructure to promote access to virtual care.

There is research supporting the financial value of telemedicine, which can be used to improve upon inpatient and outpatient care delivery by promoting blended in-person and virtual care which creates the optimal safety profile while reducing healthcare costs.

5.2.1 Hospital-Based Care

1. Telemedicine based cardiovascular ICU care is already used in approximately 15% of the beds across the United States [5]. Telemedicine ICU care leads to a decreased length of stay, reduced mortality rate and increased quality of patient care while financially benefiting the hospital.
2. Remote inpatient consults have long been used in rural and underserved areas [6] and expanded in 2020 in many countries to allow continued comprehensive high quality cardiovascular patient care during the pandemic, while also preserving revenue generation and fiscal health.
3. Pre-hospital care from the home or ambulance prior to the patient's arrival in a hospital is a growing use of telemedicine which has demonstrated cost savings [7, 8].
4. Telemedicine promotes physician wellness and engagement, thereby decreasing burnout associated patient safety errors and decreased patient satisfaction. Costs associated with staff turnover, lost revenue from decreased productivity, and financial risk with burnout-related lower quality of care highlight the financial need for cardiovascular telemedicine [9].
5. Physicians and practices also benefit from decreased travel time to rural and outlying clinic locations, improving strategic implementation of brick-and-mortar clinics with increased physician time efficiency.

5.2.2 Outpatient Care

1. Pacemaker and defibrillator surveillance based on remote monitoring is well established to be safe, efficient and cost effective while also reducing hospital visits in the long term [10, 11]. Implantable devices also provide meaningful longitudinal patient data while increasing practice revenue [12].

2. Physicians in outpatient settings can interpret remote patient monitoring data and other store and forward type data gathered from implantable devices, and can bill chronic care E&M codes and remote patient monitoring codes [13]. Mobile applications for telemedicine evaluation of atrial fibrillation was also recently developed for outpatient follow up [14].
3. Limited echocardiography by nurses in an outpatient heart failure clinic supported by interpretation by an out-of-hospital cardiologist, has been found to be feasible and reliable when using tele-echocardiography in a heart-failure clinic [15].
4. Post-discharge remote patient monitoring (RPM) enables early discharge and avoids readmissions and associated penalties [16]. Virtual cardiac rehabilitation has demonstrated improvement in exercise capacity, improves cholesterol levels & diet quality in a 16 week randomized controlled trial [17].
5. Telemedicine improves outpatient access by helping patients overcome barriers including travel limitations, time off from work, and childcare, thereby benefiting lower socioeconomic groups, primary child caregivers and the elderly [18].

5.2.3   TeleCardiology in the Home

Another new location that impacts how cardiologists practice telemedicine is the home (See Home Hospital Case). There is a growing awareness about work from home options which impacts physician quality-of-life, burnout and satisfaction. If physicians have less burnout and have more flexible hours because they can work at home, this provides an opportunity for them to see more patients or be more efficient which will translate directly into increased E&M billing. This is additional revenue to the physician's office or the hospital. Most important is maintaining a healthy and efficient workforce with low turnover. Staff recruitment, unplanned time off work due to burnout and inefficiency are financial stressors to outpatient offices and hospitals alike.

There is enough justification to be made for investing in physician wellness and engagement. Increased physician burnout is associated with higher physician turnover, and decreased productivity which can lead to lost revenue. In addition, hospitals see more patient safety errors and decreased patient satisfaction. Costs associated with turnover, lost revenue associated with decreased productivity, as well as financial risk with burnout and lower quality of care highlight the financial need for cardiovascular telemedicine [9].

One important consideration about location-based telemedicine is the expense of providing the telemedicine service as the entire financial equation is not entirely based on revenue. Telemedicine involves "tele" technology which has a capital expenses and also an operational expense. The telemedicine systems and the endpoints such as echo machines that gather the data all have communication needs, are depreciated overtime and need routine maintenance. The cost of implementing telemedicine solutions and maintaining them must be added to the value equation; typically they are paid for by a hospital or outpatient office.

An incomplete telemedicine technology implementation may result in low provider efficiency, duplicate patient records, or more technical challenges that lead to less productivity and greater maintenance expense. This would reduce clinical revenue and increase operational expense, both unfavorable for the net value for cardiologists. Therefore, the clinical design and implementation of the technology is critical.

One favorable factor about technology location is that the consumer-electronics market has enabled patients to purchase their own phones, wireless plans, computers and broadband plans that minimize the financial outlay for hospitals and outpatient offices for home telemedicine. In essence much of the expense for patients at home is "free" which is a major benefit for scaling all types of home-based telemedicine for cardiovascular care.

In summary, the connectivity and integration of telemedicine from the provider side has a real expense which is partially offset by consumers handing the cost of their endpoints. This creates a valuable future for scaling telemedicine for quality and other key clinical outcomes within a viable business model.

Practice Logistics to Support Financial Value (United States)
Practices must develop standardized front-end registration processes for telehealth patients in addition to in-person appointments. Demographic and insurance coverage verification using eligibility software can help maximize reimbursement. Addition of new networks to your practice which align with virtual care models may also be financially beneficial. CMS publishes a list of currently approved telehealth codes and The American Medical Association (AMA) compiles the CPT handbook, in which the "starred appendix" includes those codes that are telehealth eligible. National and local telehealth policies should be reviewed routinely as they will likely change over the next several years. These policies may affect licensing and credentialing requirements. As a best practice, to understand state-specific policies, providers can check the Center for Connected Health Policy State Telehealth Laws and Reimbursement Policies Report [19].

5.3   Stakeholder Based View of Cardiovascular Telemedicine Care

There is a second way to view telemedicine financial value for cardiovascular care, and that is from the perspective of the healthcare stakeholders. The key stakeholders include providers, payers, and patients. Although there are commonalities seen by location it is worthwhile seeing the care of cardiovascular telemedicine using the perspective of these primary stakeholders to tease out nuances and specific quality and economic advantages.

5.3.1 Stakeholders: Cardiologists

Healthcare providers, and cardiologists in particular, benefit financially from using telemedicine when caring for their patients as was seen in the location perspectives described above. This group of providers also includes advanced practice providers, nurses and allied health professionals. Traditional face-to-face visits can be replaced to a significant degree with telemedicine, and in the setting of Covid telemedicine may be the only modality to reach out to and provide clinical care for patients. The main challenge with routine at home telemedicine for cardiologists is the inability to listen to heart tones, but not every examination requires such data such as a routine blood pressure or medication symptom evaluation. There are peripherals and digital stethoscopes that can transmit virtual heart tones but they can be expensive and or require pairing with a phone. The capabilities and less-expensive such peripherals are emerging and may become commoditized in the near future.

If telemedicine care is able to increase compliance with patient visits, one would expect to see better quality of care and more E&M revenue captured. Yet, there can also be technical challenges with patients setting up video call software on their phones or working with remote monitoring which may slow down providers and create delays in clinics. These two facts point to a need to educate patients and providers with training and marketing materials to ensure a value-based deployment of telemedicine.

Many cardiologists perform procedures such as implanting pacemakers, implanting defibrillators, and stents during angiograms. Procedural physicians have to do a routine post-procedural evaluation of incisions and basic functionality with symptom checking. As has been seen with surgeons, this type of post-procedure or care can routinely be handled with telemedicine video visits to the home. This has significant benefits to the patients because they do not have to travel. It also impacts physician clinical efficiency as they post-procedure patients do not have to be roomed, get vital signs, and consume staff time. This typically results in more streamlined outpatient clinical operations and saves face to face time for new patients and thus new revenue.

Telemedicine also is in the emerging stage of being used to capture new patients, especially those from a wide geographical range. Meeting a new patient virtually prevents driving and expands a cardiologist's outreach geography. An in-person new visit may be difficult for a variety of social or geographical reasons for patients to come for multiple face-to-face clinic visits before or after procedures. Therefore, telemedicine enables cardiologists to expand their practice without the inefficiency of driving. There are also telemedicine pre-procedural services that evaluate patients beforehand to ensure the procedures are successful, the patients are appropriate for a procedure, and that the procedure is not canceled. With procedures, there should not be cancellations or unnecessary delays because of the negative safety implications and financial impact.

As cardiologists are rated by patients using vehicles such as Press-Gainey scores or CHAPS scores, they are held accountable for post-procedural or post-hospital care. Using technology such as remote patient monitoring and video visits to increase routine access without driving can prevent readmissions or early transfers back from nursing homes. In other words, telemedicine is a risk mitigation strategy and a patient satisfaction strategy that impacts reimbursement and provider ratings. Patients are favorably responding to telemedicine and the avoidance of unnecessary driving.

As discussed above, burnout with physicians is becoming commonplace, and therefore if a hospital or a practice group is trying to recruit a cardiologist to join them, offering telemedicine is essential [20]. Giving doctors flexible schedules that facilitate individual styles of practice can reduce burnout and may be more feasible with telemedicine [21]. Telemedicine offers the flexibility of work from home or other strategies to prevent burnout. Telemedicine based employee assistance programs or employer health clinics will result in a healthier and more productive workforce, directly tied to bottom-line financial performance.

Physicians, especially those in private practice and those in large academic medical centers may have to drive to multiple clinics to cover sufficient geography for referrals and recruiting procedures. Driving wastes valuable time and also incurs travel expenses. Therefore, using telemedicine to engage or replace remote clinics strategically is a useful and efficient way to cover or expand a cardiologist's geography.

Therefore, telemedicine can offer a wide array of benefits for providers from reducing travel time, a better quality of life, expanded patient catchment arê, and more efficient clinics. The diverse nature of telemedicine from the providers' perspective has made it challenging to quantify the exact bottom line of the financial impact. Over time, analytics and finance teams focusing on telemedicine will start better to quantify the financial performance for the cardiology community. Inherently and intuitively, telemedicine adds economic value in its current form, and it will only increase in value over time.

5.3.2   Stakeholders: Payers

Payers are one of the most important stakeholders when discussing telemedicine's financial advantages when taking care of patients or members who have cardiovascular diseases (See Medical Diagnoses using Remote Patient Monitoring). Payers represent a critical waypoint between employers and front-line healthcare. Payers also offer care delivery methodologies by their care teams such as pharmacists or care managers who interact directly with members to promote health and wellness. Payers can impact the financial landscape of telemedicine through payment policies, benefit design, sales channels, government bid process, and, more specifically, to third-party payers how they manage their Medicare advantage.

Payers directly control the financing of telemedicine through policies that dictate reimbursement for telemedicine services. They also contract individually with the

Medical Diagnoses using Remote Patient Monitoring

Medical diagnoses involving remote monitoring are ideal for payer supported virtual care

1. Asynchronous text messages improve glycemic control in patients with diabetes mellitus and coronary heart disease [22].

2. Remote clinical services augment outpatient and inpatient cardiovascular care, while favorably impacting cost [14].

3. Telemedicine models assist self-management of chronic CVD risk factors including glycemic control, weight and blood pressure reduction and increase in physical activity [23].

4. Mobile health use reduces risk of rehospitalization and clinical adverse events in patients with atrial fibrillation compared with usual care [24].

5. Home blood-pressure telemonitoring among adults in the US with uncontrolled hypertension, a 1 year intervention led to over 4 years of target BP measurements [25].

delivery side of healthcare and negotiate rates that include telemedicine services. Payers also help manage risk, especially with chronic diseases within their member cohort, using care managers. These teams can impact the total cost of care, unplanned utilization of care, and ancillary authorization. All of this directly affects the financial advantages and value of telemedicine care for cardiovascular patients. How they work with physician groups, hospitals, or the network at large through telemedicine services can have a significant impact on their medical spending across all business lines.

The Covid epidemic in particular highlighted the use of telemedicine when CMS expanded the codes for the use of telemedicine. Their forward leaning view was important to show the use of telemedicine for traditional E&M visits and in risk arrangements.

Payers also are looking to utilize niche telemedicine solutions for particular diseases such as COPD, diabetes, and heart failure that tend to be focused on remote monitoring solutions. For example, using asynchronous text messages improved glycemic control in patients with diabetes mellitus and coronary heart disease [22]. These telemedicine solutions help to help manage costs for those high spend patients and also coordinate aspects of their care such as medication reconciliation or social determinants of health. Companies such as Livongo offer a suite of remote clinical services that could augment outpatient or inpatient cardiovascular care, and overall could favorably impact the spend on these patients. Many chronic diseases have ineffective management contributing to increased health care. Remote patient monitoring RPM can an effective tool for assisting in the self-management of chronic CVD risk factors like diabetes as shown by the Mississippi Diabetes Telehealth Clinical Care model [23].

Another key area for payers is access to care for their members, and clearly telemedicine is one of the critical new tools to provide virtual access. The other traditional options of face to face clinics and inpatient care are typically expensive and can be difficult to control the unplanned and total spend. Synchronous audio-video telemedicine consults can take care of patients remotely and avert more expensive care settings and decrease costs [26].

Even if the patient stays at home, visiting nurses can drive to the patient's house which is still episodic and leverages E&M billing which is a cost accelerator. So the ability for telemedicine to provide access to patients at home or in other remote locations including care facilities is very important for care coordination, chronic disease management, and cost avoidance.

There have been challenges for the payer community in deploying telemedicine and their constant focus on financial value, and one area is the evolution of RPM. For congestive heart failure patients there is real promise for RPM, yet to date there are not the financial returns that would drive long term payer financing mechanisms put in place behind it. On the other hand, a recent study of Mobile Health technology use found reduced risks of rehospitalization and clinical adverse events in patients with Atrial fibrillation with it compared with usual care [24]. A good portion of this initial literature is likely due to early operational models and evolution of the RPM technology, but nonetheless there remains the promise that the RPM early warning system should help to provide value to the payers and help the patients avoid the care and financial challenges of unplanned care.

Third-party pears in the United States are also very cognizant of their star ratings and their health effectiveness and data information set (HEIDS). Star ratings are impacted by HEDIS scores and there is real hope that telemedicine can help close HEDIS gaps to increase scores and thus revenue. As payer quality becomes more dependent on subjective feedback, the member's convenient access to care using telemedicine should favorably impact those quality metrics and eventually revenue. For example, home blood-pressure telemonitoring among adults with uncontrolled hypertension, a substantial percent of all hypertensives in the USA, showed that after 1 year after intervention, BP remained significantly better, and didn't return to "usual" levels for over 4 years [25].

The largest payer in the US is the federal government, CMS, which has been supporting telehealth and expanding its support through increased codes and opportunities surrounding COVID. On March 172,020 CMS announced temporary telemedicine codes building upon the regulatory flexibilities granted under the President's emergency declaration allowing beneficiaries in all areas of the country to receive telehealth services, including at their home through a new waiver in Section 1135(b) of the Social Security Act. This explicitly allows the Health Secretary to authorize use of telephones that have audio and video capabilities for the furnishing of Medicare telehealth services during the COVID public health emergency.

Even before the COVID pandemic, CMS was expanding the number of codes for reimbursement for RPM and the ability to conduct remote telemedicine visits using traditional E&M coding in the US. CMS and the administrator are openly supporting telemedicine. The Wall Street Journal quoted Seema Verma, head of CMS, saying "the Genie's out of the bottle" alluding to the COVID pandemic causing telemedicine to escape from its dormant confined state into an accelerated larger form [27]. With the COVID pandemic, the telemedicine landscape shifted from a nice to have feature to mission critical with financial value as the most important driver of its continued growth.

Urgent care issues addressed with on-demand telemedicine and behavioral health were adopted early in the US payer community for reimbursement. However since 2020, the payer community, through multiple and overlapping strategies, are seeing the financial value of longitudinal cardiovascular telemedicine for prevention, chronic disease management and early identification of acute cardiovascular needs and putting in place high-level financial controls to drive its expansion and value.

5.3.3 Stakeholders: Patients

There are multiple ways that patients themselves benefit financially from telemedicine when they have cardiovascular diseases. One of the most common ways is not having to travel to the clinic. Patients with cardiovascular disease typically require longitudinal follow-up, short interval follow up after procedures or routine medication adjustments. When patients have to travel, there is the cost of gas, tolls, parking, and meals, not to mention time off work through lost wages or having to pay for childcare. Older patients also could have a difficult time driving, and therefore have to pay someone to drive them or find a relative or friend who also has to take time off work to provide transportation. The cost-benefit of telemedicine has been recognized as it avoids the expense and hassle of patient travel.

Also, as patients now have high deductible accounts through employers and payers and are more at risk for their health; having access to care can be less expensive at times if they engage the healthcare system virtually. Many payers offer lower copays for virtual first services, which directly reduces the expense of seeking healthcare. Patients can also get lower-cost advice about care options using telemedicine before incurring high-cost and high-deductible in-person services.

The most important part of patients using telemedicine is receiving high-quality care for health and well care. Still, there are undoubtedly direct avoided costs that can be of significant cumulative value for patients who require longitudinal cardiac care such as patients with complex heart failure to those with uncomplicated hypertension who require medication adjustments. It is easier to use RPM and a home blood pressure cuff then to travel several hours every month or two to keep their blood pressure checked and medication adjusted.

5.4 Summary

Telemedicine is now a foundational element of cardiovascular care delivery and benefits all healthcare stakeholders. Telemedicine impacts the entire spectrum of care delivery including consumer engagement, hospital based ancillary care, and home, outpatient, ICU and consultative care. Payers now look to telemedicine for access, care management and value. Over time, if quality and cost analyses are set up correctly, the field of cardiology will efficiently use telemedicine to optimize clinical and financial value for cardiologists, hospitals, payers, and most importantly, patients. We have reached a crucial point in telemedicine where virtual activity must be based on financial models with a sound economic underpinning.

References

1. Watson AR, Wah R, Thamman R. The value of remote monitoring for the COVID-19 pandemic. Telemed J E Health. 2020;26(9):1110–2. https://doi.org/10.1089/tmj.2020.0134.
2. Duggal R, Brindle I, Bagenal J. Digital healthcare: regulating the revolution. BMJ. 2018;360:k6.
3. Fisher NDL, Fera LE, Dunning JR, Desai S, Matta L, Liquori V, Pagliaro J, Pabo E, Merriam M, MacRae CA, Scirica BM. Development of an entirely remote, non-physician led hypertension management program. Clin Cardiol. 2019;42(2):285–91. PMID: 30582181.
4. CDC. Using telehealth to expand access to essential health services during the COVID-19 pandemic. 2020. https://www.cdc.gov/coronavirus/2019-ncov/hcp/telehealth.html
5. Vranas KC, Slatore CG, Kerlin MP. Telemedicine coverage of intensive care units: a narrative review. Ann Am Thorac Soc. 2018;15(11):1256–64. https://doi.org/10.1513/AnnalsATS.201804-225CME.
6. Klein S, Hostetter M. Using telemedicine to increase access, improve care in rural communities. 2017. https://www.commonwealthfund.org/publications/newsletter-article/2017/mar/using-telemedicine-increase-access-improve-care-rural
7. Miller AC, Ward MM, Ullrich F, Merchant KAS, Swanson MB, Mohr NM. Emergency department telemedicine consults are associated with faster time-to-electrocardiogram and time-to-fibrinolysis for myocardial infarction patients. Telemed J E Health. 2020; https://doi.org/10.1089/tmj.2019.0273.
8. Menees DS, Peterson ED, Wang Y, Curtis JP, Messenger JC, Rumsfeld JS, Gurm HS. Door-to-balloon time and mortality among patients undergoing primary PCI. N Engl J Med. 2013;369:901–9. https://doi.org/10.1056/NEJMoa1208200.
9. Shanafelt T, Goh J, Sinsky C. The business case for investing in physician well-being. JAMA Intern Med. 2017;177(12):1826–32. https://doi.org/10.1001/jamainternmed.2017.4340.
10. Watanabe E, Yamazaki F, Goto T, Asai T, Yamamoto T, Hirooka K, Sato T, Kasai A, Ueda M, Yamakawa T, Ueda Y, Yamamoto K, Tokunaga T, Sugai Y, Tanaka K, Hiramatsu S, Arakawa T, Schrader J, Varma N, Ando K. Remote management of pacemaker patients with biennial in-clinic evaluation: continuous home monitoring in the Japanese at-home study: a randomized clinical trial. Circ Arrhythm Electrophysiol. 2020;13(5):e007734. https://doi.org/10.1161/CIRCEP.119.007734.
11. García-Fernández FJ, Asensi JO, Romero R, Lozano IF, Larrazabal JM, Ferrer JM, Ortiz R, Pombo M, Tornés FJ, Kolbolandi MM, on behalf of the RM-ALONE Trial Investigators. Safety and efficiency of a common and simplified protocol for pacemaker and defibrillator surveillance based on remote monitoring only: a long-term randomized trial (RM-ALONE). Eur Heart J. 2019;40(23):1837–46. https://doi.org/10.1093/eurheartj/ehz067.

12. Slotwiner D, Varma N, Akar JG, Annas G, Beardsall M, Fogel RI, et al. HRS Expert Consensus Statement on remote interrogation and monitoring for cardiovascular implantable electronic devices. Heart Rhythm. 2015;12(7):e69–e100.
13. Verma S Early impact of CMS expansion of Medicare telehealth during COVID-19. 2020. https://www.healthaffairs.org/do/10.1377/hblog20200715.454789/abs/
14. Linz D, Pluymaekers NAHA, Hendriks JM, on behalf of the TeleCheck-AF Investigators. TeleCheck-AF for COVID-19: a European mHealth project to facilitate atrial fibrillation management through teleconsultation during COVID19. Eur Heart J. 2020;41(21):1954–5. https://doi.org/10.1093/eurheartj/ehaa404.
15. Hjorth-Hansen AK, Andersen GN, Graven T, Gundersen GH, Kleinau JO, Mjølstad OC, Skjetne K, Stølen S, Torp H, Dalen H. Feasibility and accuracy of tele-echocardiography, with examinations by nurses and interpretation by an expert via telemedicine, in an outpatient heart failure clinic. J Ultrasound Med. 2020;39(12):2313–23. https://doi.org/10.1002/jum.15341.
16. Sharp B, Buckley C. Remote Patient Monitoring 2018: High Potential in a Shifting Landscape. KLAS. 2018 Oct 2.
17. Lear SA, Singer J, Banner-Lukaris D, et al. Randomized trial of a virtual cardiac rehabilitation program delivered at a distance via the Internet. Circ Cardiovasc Qual Outcomes. 2014;7(6):952–9. https://doi.org/10.1161/CIRCOUTCOMES.114.001230.
18. Balady GJ, Ades PA, Bittner VA, et al. Referral, enrollment, and delivery of cardiac rehabilitation/secondary prevention programs at clinical centers and beyond: a presidential advisory from the American Heart Association. Circulation. 2011;124(25):2951–60. https://doi.org/10.1161/CIR.0b013e31823b21e2.
19. ATA. Telehealth basics. 2020. https://www.americantelemed.org/resource/why-telemedicine/
20. Mehta LS, Lewis SJ, Duvernoy CS, Rzeszut AK, Walsh MN, Harrington RA, Poppas A, Linzer M, Binkley PF, Douglas PS, on behalf of the American College of Cardiology Women in Cardiology Leadership Council. Burnout and career satisfaction among U.S. cardiologists. J Am Coll Cardiol. 2019;73(25):3345–8. https://doi.org/10.1016/j.jacc.2019.04.031.
21. Panagioti M, Panagopoulou E, Bower P, et al. Controlled interventions to reduce burnout in physicians: a systematic review and meta-analysis. JAMA Intern Med. 2017;177:195–205.
22. Huo X, et al. Effects of mobile text messaging on glycemic control in patients with coronary heart disease and diabetes mellitus. A randomized clinical trial. Circ Cardiovasc Qual Outcomes. 2019; https://doi.org/10.1161/CIRCOUTCOMES.119.005805.
23. Davis TC, Hoover KW, Keller S, Replogle WH. Mississippi diabetes telehealth network: a collaborative approach to chronic care management. Telemed J E Health. 2020;26(2):184–9. https://doi.org/10.1089/tmj.2018.0334.
24. Guo Y, et al. Mobile health technology to improve care for patients with atrial fibrillation. J Am Coll Cardiol. 2020;75(13):1523–34.
25. Margolis KL, Asche SE, Dehmer SP, et al. Long-term outcomes of the effects of home blood pressure telemonitoring and pharmacist management on blood pressure among adults with uncontrolled hypertension: follow-up of a cluster randomized clinical trial. JAMA Netw Open. 2018;1(5):e181617. https://doi.org/10.1001/jamanetworkopen.2018.1617.
26. Nord G, Rising KL, Band RA, Carr BG, Hollander JE. On-demand synchronous audio video telemedicine visits are cost effective. Am J Emerg Med. 2019;37(5):890–4. https://doi.org/10.1016/j.ajem.2018.08.017. Epub 2018 Aug 7. PMID: 30100333.
27. Wall Street Journal (WSJ). The doctor will zoom you now. 2020. https://www.wsj.com/articles/the-doctor-will-zoom-you-now-11587935588

Chapter 6
Telemedicine as a Cardiovascular Center Growth Strategy: Patient Experience, Provider Satisfaction and Improved Access

Jaclyn A. Pagliaro and Ami B. Bhatt

Cardiology presents itself as the ideal specialty for developing a reproducible structure for health information technology. It is immensely data driven and most guidelines have algorithms to provide comprehensive patient care. Telemedicine enables clinicians throughout the world to continually manage large populations at a distance, rather than with episodic in-person care alone [1]. Technologies such as Bluetooth enabled devices for heart rate, blood pressure, weight, oxygen saturation and activity monitoring create real-time individual cardiac fingerprints, which provide insight for the care team.

The widespread dissemination of telemedicine also enables frequent assessment and high-touch interventions. The field of cardiac monitoring and treatment devices is one of the most advanced in the medical subspecialties. This affords clinicians with an existing framework for the mechanisms and workflow for remote data collection and analysis, as exemplified in hypertension, electrophysiology, heart failure, cardiac rehabilitation and most recently in cardio-obstetrics (Table 6.1).

6.1 Patient Experience

The National Quality Forum has three recommended domains for telehealth measures: access, experience and effectiveness. Telecardiology is effective in all three areas, and has specifically been found to reduce the rate of hospitalizations and readmissions, improve morbidity and mortality rates, cardiovascular outcomes, access and quality of life, and increase cost-effectiveness and self-management of cardiovascular disease [7].

J. A. Pagliaro (✉) · A. B. Bhatt
Corrigan Minehan Heart Center, Massachusetts General Hospital, Boston, MA, USA
e-mail: jaclyn.pagliaro@mgh.harvard.edu; abhatt@mgh.harvard.edu

© Springer Nature Switzerland AG 2021
A. B. Bhatt (ed.), *Healthcare Information Technology for Cardiovascular Medicine*, Health Informatics, https://doi.org/10.1007/978-3-030-81030-6_6

Table 6.1 Successful telemedicine implementation studies by subspecialty

Hypertension [2]	In a pilot study, patients were supplied with Bluetooth blood pressure monitors that transmitted data in real-time to their electronic medical record. They were asked to measure their blood pressure at home for one week; twice daily in the morning and evening in duplicate, prior to caffeine or taking antihypertensive medications. Then weekly BPs would be averaged and antihypertensive medication titrations were made utilizing an algorithm. In this program, control was reached in 81% of patients and in 91% of patients who were engaged in the program, in an average of 7 weeks.
Electrophysiology [3]	In a comparison study of long-distance telemedicine ICD visits and conventional in-person device clinic visits, the telemedicine group was found to have lower comorbidity burden based on the Charlson score as well as a lower proportion baseline prevalence of afib. During the median follow-up of 4.4 years, telemedicine care was found to be noninferior of all outcomes.
Heart failure [4]	When comparing a remote medication monitoring system to traditional management in heart failure patients, the use of telemedicine was associated with an 80% reduction in all-cause hospitalization and of those who were hospitalized, had a reduced length of stay when compared to the usual care arm. Objective device data also indicated 95–99% adherence rates for the telemedicine group.
Cardiac rehabilitation [5]	Cardiac rehabilitation programs have the potential to reduce morbidity and mortality in cardiac patients, while also increasing quality of life. One study found that the utilization of cardiac telerehabilitation to overcome the barriers and limitations of traditional programs. By increasing the accessibility to cardiac rehab it may increase patient volumes and adherence, decrease transportation barriers, and allow for personalized coaching and support for longer intervals of time. Remote monitoring can also also be used to track patient vitals during normal daily activities, which allows for closer clinical management.
Cardio obstetrics [6]	Obstetric ultrasonographers performed fetal echocardiograms at the patient's local clinic however, the results were given to the mother in real-time by a fetal cardiologist at a children's hospital 243 miles away. The study found that neither diagnostic quality nor patient satisfaction was hindered by the use of telemedicine. The program empowered the local clinicians, offered strong economic advantages to the patients and offered a timely, face-to-face, specialty consultation without travel.

A recent use of telemedicine that is particularly useful to cardiovascular center operations is virtual pre-admission testing and evaluation. These virtual evaluations have been found to reduce overall patient time in the inpatient setting pre-operatively and improves patient satisfaction without increasing the operative case cancellation rate [8]. Streamlining periprocedural care without the use of physical hospital space and personnel allows for timely assessment and patient preparation. Patients and families are especially appreciative of both the convenience and inclusivity of the process, allowing for fewer missed days of work periprocedurally, as well as increased caregiver involvement leading to decreased anxiety.

Table 6.2 Telemedicine utilization for pre-admission, inpatients and post-discharge follow up

Chronic care & pre-admission monitoring	The remote clinical management of outpatients allows for remote patient monitoring using wearable devices. The data collected remotely can then be used to support the decision-making process of physicians.
In-hospital telecardiology	Most applications of in-hospital telecardiology refer to real-time collaborations between small hospitals and tertiary care centers. Examples include rural hospitals consulting larger institutions for the diagnosis or exclusion of congenital heart disease in newborns, or for acute stroke management. However, since the emergence of COVID-19 in-hospital telemedicine has been increasingly used between clinicians for teleconsultations to provide comprehensive care while reducing exposure and decreasing PPE utilization.
Post-hospital follow up	Close post-discharge follow up improves outcomes and reduces readmissions and urgent care utilization in patients with heart failure, arrhythmias and implantable devices.

Source: Kruse et al. [7]

Chronic disease management with virtual visits, asynchronous questionnaires and peripheral devices is also evolving. It is no longer limited to heart failure and hypertension management but also routine outpatient care and subspecialty care including cardio-obstetrics and congenital heart disease. The challenge of an effective virtual care paradigm is building an infrastructure and developing a toolbox from which heterogeneous patient populations and provider preferences can both be met to optimize a care delivery plan (Table 6.2).

6.2   Improved Access

Between WiFi and cellular data networks, patients with cardiovascular disease have access to rapidly contact their clinicians thus removing proximity from the equation of care. Telemedicine has been shown to successfully reduce barriers to traditional modalities of care such as access to transportation, travel distance and time, lack of childcare and loss of work productivity while providing comprehensive medical care with the same or greater effectiveness [7]. The use of digital health, monitoring vitals with wearables, asynchronous screening tools, virtual visits for medical management and behavioral health are revolutionizing the delivery of care in the face of social barriers to health (Table 6.3).

Social determinants including financial barriers and access to nutritious meal plans further create challenges in implementing cardiovascular health recommendations. Engaging with patients via video and in their homes allows care teams to better understand the individual circumstances, which may influence compliance with medical and lifestyle advice. This allows personalization to create a successful healthy lifestyle partnership. The involvement of family members in discussion,

Table 6.3 Evaluating access, experience and efficacy of telemedicine implementation

	At-risk populations	International patients	Procedural patients	Urgent and emergent care
Access	– Increase access to subspecialty care – Promote continuous rather than episodic chronic disease management – Identify increasing risk earlier and intervene	– Bring tertiary care to novel populations – Create a unique growth and branding opportunity – Increase education and sharing of best practices across institutions	– Increase throughput of pre- and post-operative evaluation – Decrease readmission and ED utilization with high-touch periprocedural care – Prioritize interventional timing with virtual monitoring (RPM, asynchronous, video)	– Allow rapid assessment and triage to the correct level and location of care (ie, cardiac clinic, community ED, tertiary ED) – Aid smaller institutions and practices with urgent expert evaluation – Increase expertise of pre-hospital care delivery in the field with virtual consultation
Experience	– Decrease time and cost associated with travel to visits – Allow family participation – Increase sense of respect for patient and dismantle the physician-patient hierarchy	– Allow for consultation and world-renowned expertise – Create access in areas where healthcare is lacking – Promote continuity of care among international patients, local clinicians and remote clinical teams	– Decrease time spent periprocedurally in the hospital – Decrease discomfort of travel – Increase rapidity of access to medical expertise when health-related anxiety is peaking	– Increase sense of connection with the practice in times of need – Encourage appreciation for team based care (more easily accepted and understood in times of need) – Allow participation of family members during emergent care, at times of significant illness, or end-of-life situations

Table 6.3   (continued)

Effectiveness	– Identify barriers to care by evaluating home environment – Increase touch points through remote monitoring to treat chronic diseases that disproportionately impact these populations – Increase patient education and literacy leading to better self-advocacy and compliance	– Increase access to subspecialty expertise – Increase the diversity of the patient population receiving care – Earlier identification of disease progression to allow for improved international triage	– Ensure optimal patient preparation – Engage in close post-procedural follow up – Decrease hospital readmissions	– Streamline location of services – Offer pre-hospital clinical support – Expansion of triage capability

"kitchen tours" to discuss food availability and choices, and medication storage, organization and review are a few successful social assessments which strongly influence heart health and are more difficult to address during in-person clinic visits.

6.3   Provider Satisfaction

Physicians have to navigate a rapidly expanding medical knowledge base, increased administrative burden associated with the introduction of electronic medical records and patient portals and new regulatory requirements for patient care and maintenance of certification. In addition they face an unprecedented level of evaluation including quality metrics and improving patient satisfaction [9]. Studies have shown that decreased physician satisfaction leads to burnout, which is costly, disruptive to clinic workflows and leads to rapid turnover. This collectively negatively impacts patient access to care. As a result of the COVID-19 pandemic, clinicians are under an even more burdensome workload than normal as well as pressure due to increased total health expenditures [10]. Telemedicine may promote physician wellness and engagement thus decreasing burnout and associated deficits.

In the Cardiovascular Center, a modern growth strategy optimizes the use of in-person and virtual care to improve patient safety, outcomes and satisfaction while increasing the efficiency and quality of clinical care, reducing cost and utilization. The cardiovascular center approach to care can be divided into disease management and acute care, each focus benefiting from a unique blend of virtual, in-person and hybrid services (Fig. 6.1).

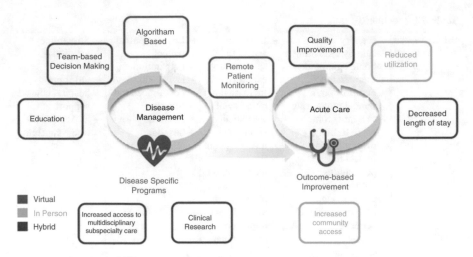

Fig. 6.1 Using fully virtual, traditional visits and hybrid models to manage chronic disease and provide acute care

6.4 Digital Health Implementation

Successful adoption of telemedicine and digital health as a growth strategy eventually requires integration at the system level of a practice, in inpatient hospital care, at skilled nursing facilities, and for at-home and clinic care. In some areas there may be remote practices and urgent care centers which require unique digital health implementation as well. Sustainable technology will require choosing a platform or application. Future iterations of virtual care may then include image interpretation, risk prediction, clinical decision support, and eventually artificial intelligence driven care. Digital health can also optimize care management by improving upon transitions of care. Payment models will have to align with provider and patient experience, clinical outcomes, and cost reduction. Telemedicine and digital health will therefore need to deliver value on these measurable endpoints. When assessing the role of digital health from chronic disease management, there are three tiers of cardiovascular patient needs which can be addressed. A majority of low-risk patients have minimal interventional needs and active surveillance can be performed in the community/at home. For the rising risk patients, more intensive at-home monitoring enables early intervention decreasing hospital resource utilization. This allows the intense care, high risk patients to benefit from timely clinic visits, diagnostic testing and procedures, and with advanced monitoring workflows, even some of these high risk patients can have an improved trajectory of safe and high quality care with continuous rather than episodic assessment (Fig. 6.2).

The IMMACULATE randomized clinical trial [11] of remote postdischarge treatment of patients with acute myocardial infarction by allied health practitioners vs standard care revealed that among low-risk patients with revascularization after myocardial infarction, remote intensive management was feasible and safe with no differences in achieved medication doses or indices of left ventricular remodeling. Additional studies in higher risk populations are underway and the massive shift to

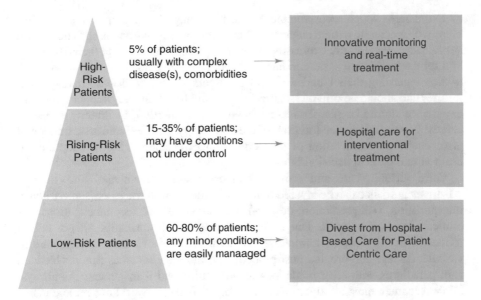

Fig. 6.2 Patient risk stratification for chronic disease management

virtual care in 2020 will likely provide additional data on the efficacy of remote monitoring and the ideal populations who will benefit from this strategy.

6.5   Guidelines and Workflows to Support Virtual Clinical Care

During the COVID pandemic, virtualizing clinical care resulted in stable quality despite moving large populations from in-person to virtual visits. The systems were built with the intention to deliver safe care and importantly, allowed in-person visits as needed. With the rapidly changing landscape of cardiovascular care and the incorporation of virtual care delivery, we need to develop agile systems, which can aid clinicians in seamlessly offering and delivering blended care. Every practice will require local guidelines regarding tele-triage of patients, identification of patient populations or diagnoses which benefit most from remote monitoring and workflows to enroll patients and acquire data. Tele-triage can include risk stratification for effective early intervention and use of digital therapeutics to enable targeted outreach to at-risk patients and optimize medical treatment. Virtual care models can aid in the adoption of guideline directed medical therapy by prompting visit frequency, medical uptitration and offering frequent at-home vital sign monitoring to allow rapid and safe medication titration and increased patient engagement compared to episodic clinic visits. Integration of clinical care guidelines and prompts can decrease loss to follow up by intentionally prompting clinician and patient to increase engagement when active management is ongoing, and otherwise allow episodic check-ins for routine stable care.

Dashboards which report remote data in a meaningful way for patients and clinicians will accelerate patient engagement and promote asynchronous chronic disease surveillance. Patients are expressing a desire to remain connected to their caregivers and for the healthcare system to harmonize fragmented care. They will need information regarding their blended virtual to in-person chronic disease management journey and should be offered technical and digital health literacy support. The user experience should be seamless to promote patient adoption, facilitating access to care while minimizing the footprint of the technology. Blended care assessment will also require standardization of data collection of accepted clinical endpoints to build virtual clinical decision tools.

Once virtual visits and remote monitoring are implemented and studied, AI-driven guidance can be layered onto care in the form of triage assistance, image interpretation, risk prediction, decision tree guided testing recommendations and clinical decision support. Diagnoses including atrial fibrillation, heart failure reduced ejection fraction, chronic secondary prevention of atherosclerotic cardiovascular disease and pre and post-procedural evaluation are areas ripe for blended care paradigms with clear guidelines for evaluation and management. As always, clinical acumen must be superimposed on any virtual care workflow, remote monitoring mechanism or AI driven decision aid.

When considering a digital health strategy for cardiovascular center growth, establishing goals and then the tools to accomplish those goals is essential. Access to high quality patient care, patient, clinician and community education and presence are all necessary in a growth strategy (Fig. 6.3). In the era of digital

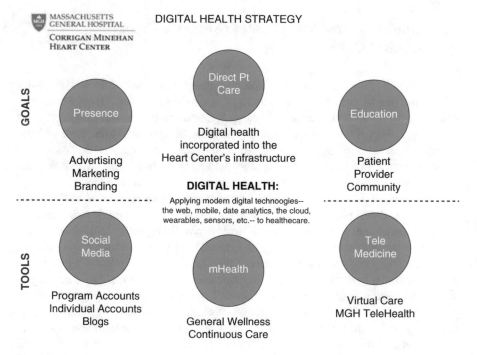

Fig. 6.3 Digital health strategy

education and literacy, telemedicine and mobile health are also accompanied by social media as a platform for patient and clinician education, entrepreneurship, and industry interaction. The skill sets needed to navigate these varied facets of the cardiovascular center footprint require multidisciplinary coordination across clinical, administrative and technology teams with a clear shared vision to engender success.

6.6   Quality Measures in Virtual Care

Telemedicine is now the fastest growing modality of healthcare delivery. It is our responsibility in the healthcare industry to ensure timely, effective, equitable and patient-centered care. This responsibility lies with the digital technology companies, their investors, hospital systems, payors, clinical teams and the patients.

As telemedicine continues to be integrated into cardiovascular care models, a comprehensive understanding of outcomes and expectations, from the clinicians' and patients' perspective, is required to advance care provision. Blended care challenges the concept of quality of virtual care as not all individuals will use the same ratio of virtual and in-person care. This reminds us that virtual care cannot be considered as an isolated mechanism of care delivery and therefore quality measures need to account for the spectrum of care from asynchronous to synchronous at a distance to in-person care. Importantly, the implementation of sustainable, virtual and in-person blended care requires that quality measures, backed by data, must extend beyond patient adoption and experience.

Practices must determine the high-priority goals for blended care implementation and create quality measures to assess achievement of those endpoints. Assessment of variables including access and compliance have already begun, however longevity and quality of life in cardiovascular patients requires assessment of mortality, disease progression and hospital admissions. Identifying quality metrics to specifically address patients with high resource utilization is a pressing clinical and financial healthcare challenge where telehealth may be leveraged to address social determinants of health and co-morbidity progression in addition to cardiac disease management.

Once priority goals are identified, the methods of evaluating virtual visits, asynchronous care and digital health data streams must be defined. National efforts by cardiovascular societies will be essential in standardizing an approach to evaluating effective telemedicine strategies. Drivers of optimization for synchronous and asynchronous care include the quality of data, contextualizing data, trends of data, and building intelligence to create relevant data interpretation. Optimal inputs to evaluate blended care include experiential, clinical and utilization metrics. Validated instruments like patient reported outcomes (PROs) which report the status of a patient's health condition without any interpretation by the patient's clinician [12] could be the first metric to transition to digitized models and be administered broadly to patients receiving virtual care. In heart failure, PROs are incredibly predictive of quality of life and outcomes and even if a patient is not involved in digital care, the PRO could be delivered digitally.

Advances in digital technology can improve clinical workflows and drive patient empowerment [13]. Clinical workflows can now include assessment with remote patient monitoring to now allow daily vital signs and medication adherence to improve clinical insights into the success of treatment plans (Fig. 6.4). Patient empowerment will increase as clinicians and patients can use these parameters to collaborate to improve engagement strategies and devise comprehensive cardiovascular care plans. Digital devices which generate automated alerts for patients will further involve them in their care and make them responsible for their own data. Collaborations between cardiovascular centers and industry will certainly accelerate the adoption of new technologies. The inclusion of patient advocacy groups will increase dissemination and adoption. Hospital patient family advisory committees should be rapidly introduced to cardiovascular center goals and strategies around digital health for active feedback, while associations with national advocacy organizations such as the American Heart Association, Marfan Foundation, Adult Congenital Heart Association and others should also incorporate their leadership and membership in the digital transformation of cardiovascular care delivery. Subspecialty care programs can serve as opportunities to closely examine the use cases, patient and provider engagement and downstream quality, outcome and financial metrics in telemedicine based blended care.

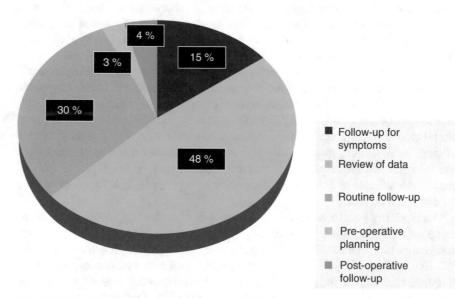

Fig. 6.4 Use cases for video visits in the MGH ACHD multidisciplinary program prior to COVID-19

Long term, the establishment of cardiovascular care delivery registries at large centers will enable quality assessment of digital tools, rapid iterations of care delivery models and opportunities for research and publication. Such registries will also aid in creating dashboards to ensure equitable access and care provision in the community. In the near-term to support clinicians and patients, vetted assessments of existing digital health platforms and products, perhaps with consideration of integration for a select few, will lessen the burden on the Cardiovascular center physician from feeling isolated in the transition to blended care. Lastly, the strategic mission of any cardiovascular center will now benefit from identifying the role of (and barriers to) telemedicine and digital health integration in emerging models of patient care and clinical research.

6.7 Conclusion

Telemedicine will undoubtedly be integrated in the future of cardiovascular healthcare delivery. The utilization of telecardiology can lessen physician burnout, disassemble the physician-patient hierarchy and allow patients to more rapidly meet their cardiovascular goals. Remote monitoring can also enhance chronic cardiac disease management and decrease the rate of hospital admissions thus reducing the overall cost of healthcare. Telemedicine increases the accessibility of care, efficiency of management and decreased utilization of resources, overcoming barriers to address social determinants of health.

The major goal for a cardiovascular center is to create an agile infrastructure to incorporate virtual care into the existing in-person workflows. In some areas, such as electrophysiology, the transition may be smooth and require minimal change based on the previous utilization of remote monitoring. Similarly, heart failure programs have already begun to optimize asynchronous and synchronous care, preventing readmissions, addressing disease progression early in its course, and significantly improving patient quality of life and satisfaction. In areas significantly dependent on the physical exam, such as valve programs, there will be a blend of remote and in-person care, a clear advantage to pre- and post-procedural virtual access, and the need to build out digital stethoscopes and remote detection of atrial fibrillation, for example. For rare diseases including adult congenital heart disease, telemedicine has increased access to specialized care and improved patient engagement.

For all of these circumstances, the diagnostic accuracy of telehealth applications, the ability to obtain actionable information to inform decision making and systems to communicate among teams and with patients in a timely manner will impact the cardiovascular center's success with virtual care delivery. The reward is extensive, with increased patient and clinician satisfaction and a proactive, equitable, personalized system of cardiovascular care delivery.

Case Study

STAT: A Digital Tool for Saving Lives at the Bedside

By Andrew L. Chu, MD, MPH, Joshua C. Ziperstein, MD, Blake A. Niccum, MD, Melvin G. Joice, MD, Eric M. Isselbacher, MD, MHCDS, Jared Conley, MD, PhD, MPH

Background

Hospitals have standardized protocols for inpatient clinicians to follow when confronting medical emergencies that carry a high risk of morbidity and mortality. Since these high acuity events (e.g. STEMI, stroke, airway emergency) occur with relatively lower frequency, clinician familiarity with workflows to expedite diagnostic and therapeutic interventions is often not fully optimized. These life-saving protocols can be difficult to access while caring for an acutely decompensating patient at the bedside, since they are often contained within e-mails or intranet websites. Although this has always been problematic during normal day-to-day operations, it was exacerbated by the COVID-19 pandemic.

Problem

In April 2020, Massachusetts General Hospital (MGH) had the highest number of COVID-19 confirmed admissions in Massachusetts. In order to accommodate this significant surge in patient volume, hospital leaders transformed existing clinical spaces into COVID-19 floors. These units were staffed by existing internal medicine (IM) staff as well as redeployed clinicians from other specialties (e.g. primary care, pediatrics, radiology). These redeployed clinicians had a wide range of depth and experience in mobilizing and working together with the MGH specialty teams that help manage these low-frequency, high acuity medical emergencies. The hospital, therefore, recognized the need for a tool that could empower all surge clinicians with rapid and reliable access to MGH-specific protocols to best manage these emergencies while at the bedside (Fig. 6.5).

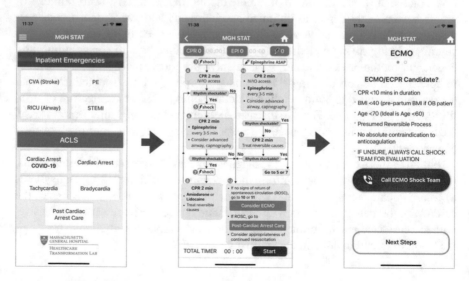

Fig. 6.5 MGH STAT Cardiac Arrest COVID-19 Pathway (2020 Launch Version)

Solution

Physician innovators within the Healthcare Transformation Lab (HTL), a MGH innovation center, and the Department of Medicine worked together to develop a mobile application, named STAT, that they could build and launch quickly across the hospital. They conducted informal surveys on which protocols clinicians would prefer to have rapid access to (e.g. STEMI, PE, CVA, ACLS, PE, respiratory failure). Subsequently, the project leaders went through a design thinking process that involved rapid cycles of ideation, prototyping, and testing, with feedback elicited from all stakeholders, including department heads, to continuously improve the product during each cycle. The final version of STAT had 9 emergency protocols, the ability to page and call consultants directly (e.g. activate Cath lab, ECMO), and various code-running features. The Hospital Incident Command System (HICS) leadership labelled the STAT app a high-priority project, so it was launched broadly to become available to all surge clinicians. The tool has been downloaded by hundreds of clinicians, and 100% of surveyed physicians recommended STAT for clinical use. As of April 2021, a year later, the mobile app continues to enjoy regular use.

Conclusion

This case report showcases the effectiveness of STAT as a digital adjunct for managing bedside emergencies. Physician innovators identified a pressing need, and they worked with stakeholders to rapidly design, develop, and deploy a tool that could be scaled throughout the hospital. Although STAT was invaluable during the worst of the pandemic, it continues to be used regularly during normal day-to-day operations. This example illustrates how clinicians identified and rapidly addressed a large-scale problem by leveraging the power of digital health.

Appendix: STAT User Experience Questionnaire

MGH STAT App Survey

MGH STAT is a native iphone app that was released through the MGB app catalog in 4/2020. The goal of the app is to help doctors manage acute, life threateining emergencies at the bedside, In this survey. we hope to solicit feedback from MGH residents and attending who have downloaded the app.

I would recommend the MGH STAT app to others, especialy interns, junior residents, and non medicine attendings.

	1	2	3	4	5	
Strongly Disagree	○	○	○	○	○	Strongly Agree

I think the MGH STAT app is easy to use.

	1	2	3	4	5	
Strongly Disagree	○	○	○	○	○	Strongly Agree

I think the MGH STAT app helps doctors manage acute life threacening emergencies (ACLS, airway crisis CVA, PE, STEM) at the bedside.

	1	2	3	4	5	
Strongly Disagree	○	○	○	○	○	Strongly Agree

I think the MGH STAT app helps improve patient care.

	1	2	3	4	5	
Strongly Disagree	○	○	○	○	○	Strongly Agree

I think apps like MGH STAT would be useful at other hospitals and healthcare settings.

	1	2	3	4	5	
Strongly Disagree	○	○	○	○	○	Strongly Agre

References

1. Bhatt, A & Pagliaro, J. The ideal model for telemedicine: digital health care delivery. 2020. https://advances.massgeneral.org/cardiovascular/article.aspx?id=1195
2. Fisher NDL, Fera LE, Dunning JR, Desai S, Matta L, Liquori V, Pagliaro J, Pabo E, Merriam M, MacRae CA, Scirica BM. Development of an entirely remote, non-physician led hypertension management program. Clin Cardiol. 2019;42(2):285–91. PMID: 30582181.
3. Turakhia MP. Telemedicine for management of implantable defibrillators: lessons learned and a look toward the future. Circ Arrhythm Electrophysiol. 2017;10(9):e005728.
4. Hale TM, Jethwani K, Kandola MS, Saldana F, Kvedar JC. A remote medication monitoring system for chronic heart failure patients to reduce readmissions: a two-arm randomized pilot study. J Med Internet Res. 2016;18(5):e91.
5. Peters RJG. Cardiac rehabilitation and telemedicine (and COVID-19). Neth Hear J 2020;28(9):441–2.
6. Cuneo BF, Olson CA, Haxel C, Howley L, Gagnon A, Benson DW, et al. Risk stratification of fetal cardiac anomalies in an underserved population using telecardiology. Obstet Gynecol. 2019;134(5):1096–103.
7. Kruse CS, Soma M, Pulluri D, Nemali NT, Brooks M. The effectiveness of telemedicine in the management of chronic heart disease—a systematic review. JRSM Open. 2017;8(3):2054270416681747.
8. Mullen-Fortino M, Rising KL, Duckworth J, Gwynn V, Sites FD, Hollander JE. Presurgical assessment using telemedicine technology: impact on efficiency, effectiveness, and patient experience of care. Telemed J E Health. 2019;25(2):137–42. https://doi.org/10.1089/tmj.2017.0133.
9. Shanafelt TD, Dyrbye LN, West CP. Addressing physician burnout: the way forward. JAMA. 2017;317(9):901–2.
10. Moazzami B, Razavi-Khorasani N, Moghadam AD, Farokhi E, Rezaei N. COVID-19 and telemedicine: immediate action required for maintaining healthcare providers well-being. J Clin Virol. 2020;126:104345.
11. Chan MY, KWL K, Poh S-C, et al. Remote postdischarge treatment of patients with acute myocardial infarction by allied health care practitioners vs standard care: the IMMACULATE randomized clinical trial. JAMA Cardiol. 2020;30:e206721. https://doi.org/10.1001/jamacardio.2020.6721.
12. Moons P, Luyckx K, Thomet C, Budts W, Enomoto J, Sluman MA, et al. Patient-reported outcomes in adults with congenital heart disease following hospitalization (from APPROACH-IS). Am J Cardiol. 2021;145:135–42.
13. Fasing K, Lathkar-Pradhan S, Bray K. Telemedicine: enabling patients with arrhythmias in self-care behaviors. Clin Case Rep Open Access. 2020;3(3):166.
14. "IHME: COVID-19 Projections." Institute for Health Metrics and Evaluation. https://covid19.healthdata.org/united-states-of-america.
15. Shanafelt T, Ripp J, Trockel M. Understanding and addressing sources of anxiety among health care professionals during the COVID-19 pandemic. JAMA. Published online 7 Apr 2020. doi:https://doi.org/10.1001/jama.2020.5893
16. Keesara S, Jonas A, Schulman K. Covid-19 and Health care's digital revolution. N Engl J Med. 2020; https://www.nejm.org/doi/full/10.1056/NEJMp2005835
17. Oxley TJ, Mocco J, Majidi S, et al. Large-vessel stroke as a presenting feature of Covid-19 in the young. N Engl J Med. 2020;382(20):e60. https://doi.org/10.1056/NEJMc2009787.
18. Clerkin Kevin J, Fried Justin A, Jayant R, et al. COVID-19 and cardiovascular disease. Circulation. 2020;141(20):1648–55. https://doi.org/10.1161/CIRCULATIONAHA.120.046941.
19. Baldi E, Sechi GM, Mare C, et al. Out-of-hospital cardiac arrest during the Covid-19 outbreak in Italy. N Engl J Med. Published online 29 Apr 2020. doi: https://doi.org/10.1056/NEJMc2010418

20. Bikdeli B, Madhavan MV, Jimenez D, et al. COVID-19 and thrombotic or thromboembolic disease: implications for prevention, antithrombotic therapy, and follow-up. J Am Coll Cardiol. Published online 17 Apr 2020. doi:https://doi.org/10.1016/j.jacc.2020.04.031
21. Edelson DP, Sasson C, Chan PS, et al. Interim guidance for basic and advanced life support in adults, children, and neonates with suspected or confirmed COVID-19: From the Emergency Cardiovascular Care Committee and get with the Guidelines®-Resuscitation Adult and Pediatric Task Forces of the American Heart Association in Collaboration with the American Academy of Pediatrics, American Association for Respiratory Care, American College of Emergency Physicians, The Society of Critical Care Anesthesiologists, and American Society of Anesthesiologists: Supporting Organizations: American Association of Critical Care Nurses and National EMS Physicians. Circulation. 0(0). doi:https://doi.org/10.1161/CIRCULATIONAHA.120.047463
22. Altman M, Huang TTK, Breland JY. Design thinking in health care. Prev Chronic Dis. 2018;15:E117. Published 27 Sep 2018. doi:https://doi.org/10.5888/pcd15.180128
23. De Simone V, Guarise P, Guardalben S, Padovani N, Tondelli S, Sandrini D, et al. Telecardiology during the Covid-19 pandemic: past mistakes and future hopes. Am J Cardiovasc Dis. 2020;10(2):34–47.

Chapter 7
The Digital Transformation of Cardiovascular Clinic Workflows

Srinath Adusumalli

7.1 Introduction

Digital transformation is the process of using digital technologies to reimagine processes, culture, and in the case of healthcare, patient and provider experiences [1]. It is as much a cultural change as it is a change in the use of technology and involves a fundamental shift in the way technology is used to transform patient and provider experiences. As providers, practices, and health systems have gained familiarity with telehealth technology, digital transforming cardiovascular clinic workflows has become imperative to refining telemedical practice. From appointment scheduling, to intra-visit workflow, to checkout and follow-up care, the entire process of a cardiovascular patient-clinician visit has the potential to be transformed with the advent of broader utilization of telehealth. Rather than directly transfer in-person mechanisms of conducting a cardiovascular clinic visit to virtual formats, the transition to telehealth practice presents an opportunity to completely rethink the ways through which outpatient care is delivered. This chapter will explore how traditional cardiovascular clinic workflows can be re-engineered via the use of telehealth and related technologies, starting with a deeper dive into the process of digital transformation.

7.2 Digital Transformation

The process of digital transformation is about much more than simply moving information from analog to digital format (known as *digitization*) or even using that information to make established ways of work simpler and easier (known as

S. Adusumalli (✉)
University of Pennsylvania Health System, Philadelphia, PA, USA
e-mail: srinath.adusumalli@pennmedicine.upenn.edu

© Springer Nature Switzerland AG 2021
A. B. Bhatt (ed.), *Healthcare Information Technology for Cardiovascular Medicine*, Health Informatics, https://doi.org/10.1007/978-3-030-81030-6_7

digitalization) [1]. As opposed to digitization and digitalization, digital transformation is about fundamentally reworking processes, culture, and experiences (or creating new ones) using technology—in essence, taking advantage of technology to inform how an organization runs. The implementation of telehealth within cardiovascular clinics has presented an ideal opportunity to digitally transform those clinics. Organizations which have adopted principles from the process of digital transformation in telehealth efforts have found the following elements critical to success [2–4]:

1. Promote agility: Given the changing telehealth environment, teams need to be able to rapidly prototype, test, and iterate on workflows. This also means team members need to feel able to take risks in decision-making, not being afraid to fail (but fail fast and learn from failure).
2. Embed into the frontline: By having telehealth champions embedded in the frontline of care, those champions have been able to engage frontline stakeholders in change management around telehealth process and technology, bring back ideas for improvement in telehealth systems, and then close the loop with stakeholders once changes/improvements are made. This process allows for sustained engagement of frontline stakeholders in the process and culture change of digital transformation.
3. Develop digital competencies and fluency: Just as important as being embedded in the frontline is equipping both frontline operational and technical teams to know what is possible with, actively participate in, and advance digital transformation efforts. Digital competence "is a combination of knowledge, skills and attitudes with regards to the use of technology to perform tasks, solve problems, communicate, manage information, collaborate, as well as to create and share content effectively, appropriately, securely, critically, creatively, independently and ethically" [5]. Building digital competence for all members of the healthcare team is critically important to more not only telehealth efforts but digital transformation in general forward.
4. Build analytics infrastructure alongside telehealth tools: As the old adage goes, it is difficult to improve what can't be measured. As such, as digital workflows are built or re-engineered, opportunities should be leveraged to embed measurement tools into workflow wherever possible. Examples of this will be given further in this text.

One facet of cardiovascular telehealth practice which can directly promote and catalyze digital transformation is the selection of an appropriate telehealth platform, which we will discuss next.

Telehealth Platform Selection: *A Launching Pad for Equitable Cardiovascular Clinic Digital Transformation*

One of the most critical decisions in the digital transformation of the cardiovascular clinic is the selection of a telehealth platform. A foundational principle in this process should be that the platform enables providers and practices to reach all the patients they care for in an equitable, high-quality, and flexible yet highly reliable fashion. Given emerging evidence that variation in clinician and clinic practices may contribute to differential access to telemedical care, it is critical for a telehealth platform to offer a range of tools which promote easy, seamless, and effective telehealth workflows [6]. Ideally, given known inequities among patient populations in access to EHR-based patient portals, the telehealth platform would have the ability to be both embedded in the portal but also be used outside of interacting with a portal. Based on this, there are several elements of platform which can help advance digital transformation:

1. No requirement for patient application downloads to utilize video telehealth services: Application downloads, whether they are onto a mobile or desktop device, present a barrier to engaging in care. This is because they require knowledge of installation processes as well as recall of pieces of information such as app store passwords. Rather than relying on the download of an application (or even multiple applications as some platforms currently require), a telehealth platform should be able to facilitate visits directly in modern desktop and mobile browsers using the popular WebRTC (real-time communications) protocol [7]. This minimizes the number of steps required to engage in a telehealth encounter.
2. Integrated accessibility services: Ease of access to video and audio interpretation services is critical to ensure all patients can participate in telehealth encounters [8–10]. Several interpretation vendors now offer integrations for telehealth platforms to facilitate joining of interpreters in the patient's preferred language with 1–2 clicks. Furthermore, services such as closed captioning as well as encounter transcription should be offered directly through telehealth platforms
3. Bidirectional communication: Real-time textual communication in the perivisit period between patients and care teams is critical to the success of the process of delivering telehealth. This can be achieved directly through telehealth platform chat functionality (ideally automated/using chatbots) or even through SMS text messaging tied into the platform. This type of communication is important because it allows care teams and patients not in the same locations to quickly communicate about issues such as the provider running behind or the patient having connection difficulties. Through available cloud services (such as Microsoft Azure), these messages can even be translated into other languages.
4. Multiparty connection: Multiparty connection is critical to the successful scaling of telehealth. Of course, the patient is the most important participant in a telehealth encounter; however, virtual exam rooms created by telehealth platforms should offer the ability for other relevant parties to participate in encounters such as patient family members or, importantly, interpreter services. When used, the platform should be able to directly integrate with interpreter services in order to make it easy to engage those services.
5. Electronic health record integration: Although there are several levels of EHR integration, at the least, the telehealth platform should be able to receive appointment/encounter and basic patient information data from the EHR in

order to facilitate sending unique, secure, patient-specific virtual exam/meeting room links to patients. This should be able to be done inside of the patient portal (given integration with tools such as pre-check-in) but also outside of it via email and SMS text messaging given well documented inequities in patient portal access [11].

6. Compatibility with multiple devices: Telehealth platforms should be able to be utilized to participate in video visits from a provider perspective on a diverse array of desktop or mobile devices to provide maximal flexibility, especially when hospital-issued computers are not available. The ability to be used across multiple devices also facilitates the utilization of another device as a second screen such that a telehealth encounter can be run on, for example, a mobile device while the EHR is running on an available computer. This flexibility, must, of course be balanced with appropriate consideration towards security.

7. Virtual waiting room: Given clinical visits often do not run on time, a telehealth platform should allow patients to wait for their encounter in a virtual waiting room. Ideally, this waiting room could be customized for an organization, offering branding as well as the opportunity to deliver customized educational material or even the opportunity to engage patients through completion of patient reported outcomes instruments. This waiting room should also make clear to patients they are in the correct spot (and should wait for their clinician to join) to prevent confusion regarding appropriate location of telehealth visit.

8. Screen/image sharing: Provider and patient screen/imaging sharing is an important aspect of telehealth. Providers should be able to share screens in order to review notes as well as testing/imaging results directly with patients during an encounter. A patient should also be able to share to synchronously or asynchronously send images or video (particularly important for fields such as dermatology).

9. Telehealth analytics: Given the practice of telehealth is rapidly developing, it is critical for care teams to be able to measure and improve on how care is being delivered. This means having access to analytics from telehealth platforms in addition to the EHR. Examples of useful analytics include video and audio bitrate, hiccup rate, frame rate, patient device and OS platform, and patient location

10. Provider usability enhancements: Given interactions with patients through telehealth platforms are completely digital, those interactions should make use of the full breadth of digital video tools through the platform, including employing virtual backgrounds, synchronizing telehealth appointments directly to clinician calendars, and automatically calculating the time each participant spent in a visit. These features greatly improve the ease with which clinicians conduct visits and keep them engaged in the process of delivering telemedical care.

With a telehealth platform in place, care teams can turn to each phase of a visit to examine where workflows can be digitally transformed.

7.3   Appointment Scheduling

Traditionally, appointment scheduling for ambulatory visits has occurred either via phone call to clinics or physically in clinic itself. Virtual workflows, particularly those associated with the already digital interactions of telehealth visits, offer the opportunity to revisit that process, particularly through utilizing features common in many patient portals. Patient visit self-scheduling can be enabled through portals and can be quickly implemented, especially for patients known to a particular provider. Most portals offer the opportunity to implement self-scheduling within the context of decision trees/branching tree logic, incorporating automated criteria to help guide a patient to appropriate types of visits and visit modalities. The process of developing a visit decision tree to embed within a portal is useful as it facilitates the structuring of clinic decisions around which clinical scenarios are best suited for in-person vs. virtual encounters [12, 13]. These visit decision trees match with provider clinic templates/schedules which have embedded in-person and telehealth slots and further facilitate the process of structuring. Finally, this process allows virtual visits to be as available as in-person visits to patients and reduces the amount of friction in engaging in both in-person and virtual care (such as waiting on hold to schedule via a call center). Moving forward, self-scheduling opportunities should be available inside and outside of patient portals, given limitations in equitable access previously noted. One way to operationalize this would be by using text messaging to connect to EHR-based schedules and offer the ability to see available appointment slots, modality, and ultimately a method through which to schedule into those slots. This is not dissimilar from the ways companies in other industries, such as OpenTable in the restaurant industry, have digitally transformed their interactions with customers. Finally, historically clinicians have not been able to directly schedule appointments with patients within the EHR. With the advent of flexible telehealth encounters, which can be conducted with a moment's notice—in response to an on-call phone call for example—quick schedule workflows within the EHR should be enabled to allow patient and clinician flexibility in scheduling while maintaining downstream processes such as visit link generation, documentation, and billing.

7.4   Preparing for the Visit

Once a visit is scheduled appropriately, both the patient and the care team can prepare for it. As above, it is important that communications occur via email, SMS text message, and the patient portal when available to ensure patients can access messaging, pre-visit activities, and virtual exam room links. As soon as a visit is scheduled, the telehealth platform or EHR should be able to send an email, SMS text message, or patient portal message containing a unique, patient/encounter specific visit link to the patient along with encounter specific messaging on how to prepare for that encounter—both from a technical and clinical perspective (such as have medications and home blood pressures readings available for the visit). This is like messages sent in other industries such as airlines where customers are prepared for upcoming flights. The advantage of having a visit link available from the time of scheduling to both the patient and clinical care team is that it can be used for pre-visit interactions such as medication or medical history reconciliation. The same link as the actual visit could also be used to confirm and assist the patient with ensuring they are technically ready for their appointment. This preparatory message could be repeated in the 24–48 h leading up to an appointment. As one final confirmation, only the visit link itself could be sent automatically—ideally via SMS text message—in the minutes prior to an encounter time. This will ensure the patient has this information readily available for this encounter. Many EHRs also offer "pre-check-in" functionality that is quite like tools offered by airlines used to obtain a boarding pass prior to a flight. These should be enabled for virtual as well as in-person visits—the questionnaires included within these workflows offer the opportunity to collect nonclinical information such as updated insurance but also important telehealth-adjacent clinical information such as past history, medications, and patient-reported outcomes measurements. One final advantage of "pre-check-in" is information collected through it can directly populate appropriate EHR fields without further care team intervention.

7.5   Conducting the Visit

Once the patient arrives for their virtual visit, features of the telehealth platform discussed above can be utilized to ensure the patient and clinician conduct an effective encounter. If closed captioning or audio transcription is available via the platform and beneficial from a patient accessibility standpoint, this should be turned on at the beginning of the encounter, ideally in automated fashion as determined by accessibility preferences passed from the EHR. Bidirectional messaging is critical at this point. The patient and care team need to be able to stay in contact such that the patient is informed as to the status of their visit (i.e. is the provider running late, should they join the virtual exam room). This type of visit coordination ordinarily is expected during in-person visits but is more difficult to accomplish virtually. Especially when clinicians conduct mixed in-person and telehealth clinics, the synchronization of timing of virtual visits is key. Several organizations have found that although this communication can be carried out via a patient portal, patients are often delayed in seeing these messages. Borrowing from other industries, SMS text messaging can assist with quick, templated messages informing the patient, for example, a provider is running late and they should continue to wait in an exam room. This can also be accomplished via in-virtual room chat if offered by a telehealth platform. With regards to coordinating the activities of multiple care team members, teams (nurses, medical assistants, providers) can utilize other virtual rooms on the telehealth platform or even on widely available collaboration platforms (Microsoft Teams, for example) to help coordinate and discuss patient cases prior to providers entering a room—a virtual visit "green room" of sorts. This type of "green room" is also effective as a precepting space for trainee encounters. Providers should also not neglect to fully utilize features of telehealth platforms such as screen/content sharing during a visit—this can be a good use of telehealth encounters for the purpose of patient education. One consideration to keep in mind is that content sharing can consume additional bandwidth in addition to video/audio and as such can degrade the quality of a connection.

7.6   After the Visit

At the conclusion of the clinical encounter, it is critical that visit follow up tasks such as scheduling of downstream appointments and testing are not lost. One way to accomplish this is by having the patient remain in virtual exam room after a provider exits. An administrative staff member can then enter to guide the patient through scheduling tests and visits, like when a patient visits an in-person checkout desk. The EHR should also be able to discretely capture follow up information with regards to modality of follow up visit agreed upon through shared decision-making by the patient/clinician (i.e., in-person vs. telehealth) and expected timing of visits. This information can be queried later to ensure no follow-up activities are being lost. As mentioned above, collaboration platforms can be used to coordinate this activity among teams or alerting functionality can be built into telehealth platforms to inform other care team members when a provider has left the room. Moving into the future, this type of follow up scheduling could be done automatically via chatbot embedded in a portal or SMS text messaging if information regarding provider follow up intent is captured discretely in the EHR. Given telehealth is a relatively new vehicle for delivering care, automated mechanisms should be available either through a telehealth platform or outside of it to assess patient and provider satisfaction after a visit, immediately after a visit. This can be done with as little as one question (i.e., "How did we do today?") along with space for a comment, all delivered via SMS text message, email, or patient portal; as with many of the workflows above, this is a technique borrowed from many other industries such as retail and restaurants. The advantage of capturing this information immediately adjacent to a visit is that it can be used for near-real-time continuous quality improvement using the voice of the patient (and provider/care team) for guidance. Finally, the fact a patient was able to successfully complete a virtual visit should be captured discretely in the EHR not only for billing reasons but also for quality improvement and future visit scheduling purposes.

7.7 Conclusion

This chapter has illustrated the power of digital transformation of cardiovascular clinic technology platforms and workflows in the context of the ongoing addition of virtual channels of care to our healthcare delivery system. Just as much as a technological shift, digital transformation is a cultural one, giving care teams the opportunity to fully reimagine the care they have delivered for years with digital tools in mind. Moving forward, all members of the care team should focus on developing digital competency and fluency to help advance virtual channels of care as a method of caring for and engaging our patients.

Case
A 66-year-old female with a past medical history of hypertension, hyperlipidemia, and coronary artery disease s/p STEMI and PCI to the proximal LAD contacts your cardiovascular clinic for a follow-up appointment to discuss her antihypertensive medications. Her preferred language is Spanish as expressed by her and documented in structured fields in the EHR. She has been taking her home blood pressures and has persistently found them to be greater than >140/90 and would like to discuss next steps in management. Your clinic has implemented and refined a set of digital workflows, so is able to offer a virtual visit the next day with an advanced practice provider (APP) in your practice. The clinic EHR has an indicator that this patient has successfully participated in virtual visits previously and therefore does not need a tutorial in setting up her devices appropriately. As soon as the visit is scheduled, the patient receives an email and SMS text message-based confirmation of scheduling— these messages also contain an active visit link and instructions regarding the visit, including a request of the patient to have her blood pressure cuff and medications available for review by the provider. They are translated into Spanish given her preferred language preference. Given the appointment is the next day, the messages also have a link to pre-check-in activities within the EHR patient portal through which the patient can confirm her insurance, history, and medications. 15 min prior to her visit, the patient receives a SMS text message with a reminder of the active visit link and nudges her to join the virtual exam room—the link takes the patient directly to the exam room in a phone browser without requiring an application download. Once in the room, the patient receives a chat message that her provider is running 5 min behind, so she remains in the room waiting for your APP. This message is also translated into Spanish. Your APP joins the patient in the virtual exam room and can quickly jump into the visit as the patient has her medications and blood pressure logs available for virtual/visual review—she had also uploaded these to the EHR during the pre-check-in process. Your APP also, with two clicks, requests a Spanish interpreter to join into the visit via video—the interpreter

joins within 1 min. Based on available information, your APP starts a new anti-hypertensive medication and requests the patient obtains labs as well as another visit in 2 weeks. At the conclusion of the visit, your APP messages your administrative assistant (AA) via your clinic collaboration platform to join the virtual exam room. Your AA joins the room and schedules the patient for labs as well as a follow up visit. At the conclusion of the encounter, the patient receives a text message asking her to rate the quality of the visit, which she thought was excellent. The APP also receives a similar message to rate the quality of the telemedical encounter.

What does success look like in the digital transformation of cardiovascular care?

- Every cardiovascular clinic team member is knowledgeable and fluent in the use of available technology to advance the care of the clinic patient population.
- Virtual care is accessible to all patients in an equitable fashion.
- Available digital tools are used to reimagine and create new workflows which were not possible in the analog world.
- Information from digital encounters (including visit analytics as well as patient and provider satisfaction measures) is used to help improve the quality of future telemedical encounters.

References

1. What is digital transformation? A definition by salesforce. Salesforce.com. https://www.sales-force.com/products/platform/what-is-digital-transformation/. Accessed 9 Jan 2021.
2. Choi K, Adusumalli S, Lee K, Rosin R, Asch DA. 5 Lessons from Penn Medicine's crisis response. Harvard Business Review. Published online 22 Jun 2020. https://hbr.org/2020/06/5-lessons-from-penn-medicines-crisis-response. Accessed 9 Dec 2020
3. Digital transformation is not about technology. Harvard Business Review. Published online 13 Mar 2019. https://hbr.org/2019/03/digital-transformation-is-not-about-technology. Accessed 9 Jan 2021
4. Wechsler LR, Adusumalli S, Deleener ME, Huffenberger AM, Kruse G, Hanson CW III. Reflections on a health system's telemedicine marathon. Telemedicine Reports. 2020;1(1):2–7. https://doi.org/10.1089/tmr.2020.0009.
5. Skov A.. The digital competence wheel. https://digital-competence.eu/front/what-is-digital-competence/. Accessed 10 Jan 2021.
6. Rodriguez JA, Betancourt JR, Sequist TD, Ganguli I. Differences in the use of telephone and video telemedicine visits during the COVID-19 pandemic. Am J Manag Care. 2021;27(1):21–6. https://doi.org/10.37765/ajmc.2021.88573.
7. WebRTC. WebRTC. https://webrtc.org/. Accessed 15 Jan 2021.
8. Eberly LA, Kallan MJ, Julien HM, et al. Patient characteristics associated with telemedicine access for primary and specialty ambulatory care during the COVID-19 pandemic. JAMA Netw Open. 2020;3(12):e2031640. https://doi.org/10.1001/jamanetworkopen.2020.31640.

9. Eberly LA, Khatana SAM, Nathan AS, et al. Telemedicine outpatient cardiovascular care during the COVID-19 pandemic: bridging or opening the digital divide? Circulation. 2020;142(5):510–2. https://doi.org/10.1161/CIRCULATIONAHA.120.048185.
10. Julien HM, Eberly LA, Srinath A. Telemedicine and the forgotten America. Circulation. 2020;142(4):312–4. https://doi.org/10.1161/CIRCULATIONAHA.120.048535.
11. Digital health equity as a necessity in the 21st century cures act era | Health Care Delivery Models | JAMA | JAMA Network. https://jamanetwork.com/journals/jama/fullarticle/2766776?resultClick=1. Accessed 15 Jan 2021.
12. Croymans D, Hurst I, Han M. Telehealth: the right care, at the right time, via the right medium. NEJM Catalyst Innovations in Care Delivery. Published online 30 Dec 2020. https://catalyst.nejm.org/doi/full/10.1056/CAT.20.0564. Accessed 16 Jan 2021.
13. A hybrid model of in-person and telemedicine facilitates care delivery. MASS General advances in motion. https://advances.massgeneral.org/cardiovascular/article.aspx?id=1334. Accessed 24 Jan 2021.

Chapter 8
Optimizing Telehealth for Special Populations and Closing the Digital Divide: Addressing Social Determinants of Health in Virtual Care

Samantha Gonzalez, Ami B. Bhatt, and Jaclyn A. Pagliaro

8.1 Elderly Populations

There are certain preconceptions about the elderly and their capacity for evolving technology. While it is acknowledged that patients in the 80+ range were bred in an era of when telephone calls required an operator, they are also historically a generation of resilience and adaptability, particularly with regard to medical treatment and technology. Patients in their 80s and 90s at the time of this publication lived through development and expansion of medical advancements such as the first use of penicillin in the 1940s and the onset of routine vaccinations for disease prevention. It is important not only to understand elderly patients' existing familiarity with technology prior to recommending virtual visits, but also to frame the introduction of technology in their care and yet another medical advancement they participate in during their lifetime. Improving their confidence in their ability to use technology and the potential service it offers may position all players for success.

Patient perceptions about telemedicine can be tackled head on in the elderly. Use of the internet and other forms of communication via cellular phones, tablets, and computers have emerged as points of access and improved convenience for several instrumental activities of daily living such as shopping, using transportation, managing medications and finances at one's fingertips in a population with varying degrees of dependence, interdependence and independence which is evaluated at

S. Gonzalez
Telehealth Implementation COVID Response, Holy Cross Health, Silver Spring, MD, USA

University of Miami Internal Medicine Residency Program, Miami, FL, USA

University of Miami Miller School of Medicine, Miami, FL, USA

A. B. Bhatt · J. A. Pagliaro (✉)
Corrigan Minehan Heart Center, Massachusetts General Hospital, Boston, MA, USA
e-mail: abhatt@mgh.harvard.edu; jaclyn.pagliaro@mgh.harvard.edu

© Springer Nature Switzerland AG 2021   101
A. B. Bhatt (ed.), *Healthcare Information Technology for Cardiovascular Medicine*, Health Informatics, https://doi.org/10.1007/978-3-030-81030-6_8

least annually at medical appointments for the elderly. It may be helpful to leverage the inevitable increased utilization of real-time audio and video communication during the COVID-19 pandemic for purposes not only in the workplace, but also for many as a form of regular communication among family members and acquaintances regardless of age. We have some information about its uses in the medical space by older patients. Existing data, while limited, suggests high rates of patient satisfaction in participants over the age 65 with telemedicine models, improved confidence in technology use in those who had nursing assistance, improved cost compared to in-person alternates, and a decline in emergency room visits. Some of the biggest barriers included patient and technology based audio-visual complications, in addition to adapting to utilizing a telemedicine portal [1]. Some tips for success as seen with the palliative care population include informing patients and caregivers about telemedicine navigation tools and communication etiquette including mute function if not actively engaged in conversation, and inform patients that there are reasons you may deem an in-person evaluation necessary, such as a change in patient's clinical status, or need for cardiovascular or pulmonary exam, for example [2]. Reassuring patients who are hesitant to participate in virtual visits that in-person visits are still an option may increase their confidence in the virtual encounter.

There are clear opportunities for video visits in older adults. On the one hand, video visits can be effectively used for prescription renewals, health promotion, and advanced care planning; to limit travel for those unable to commute to clinic independently, which may prove especially helpful for patients undergoing palliative care; for routine follow-up after device implantation, such as pacemaker and defibrillators; and for care coordination among clinicians. In this model, low acuity needs can be readily achieved, and aspects of care delivery focused on cost reduction and for convenience can be enhanced. On the other hand, video visits are emerging as a potential vehicle for complex care delivery. Data from clinical trials and meta analyses of telehealth in conditions such as stroke [3] and heart failure [4] have demonstrated confidence in self-care, improvements in measures of patient reported outcomes, and in select cohorts, a lower risk of hospitalizations (stroke and HF ref. above). For example, Comin-Colet et al. investigated the role of video visits with daily assessment of signs and symptoms compared with usual face-to-face encounters on the quality of care and outcomes among an older adult cohort of heart failure patients. Compared with usual care, patients randomized to video visits (mean age 77 years, 25% identified as frail) experienced a lower risk of heart failure readmission at 6 months and conferred a lower net reduction in direct hospital costs. Although the aggregate of these data is reassuring in that there were no safety signals or untoward risks of video-based care alone, it does raise questions as to how a model of frequent video visits, or a hybrid model, can be pragmatically adopted, and if this level of non–face-to-face care is required to mitigate adverse outcomes among a high risk older adult cohort with complex diseases.

"Tele-assistance" is a model in which counseling services with different health care professionals over video is combined with remote monitoring of vital signs and functional assessments over time. De Cola et al. [5] assessed the feasibility of tele-assistance among 131 patients with multiple comorbidities (mean age 80 years,

60% in rural locations) in a design that included monthly neurophysiological and nutritional services to address cognitive needs and those factors related to anthropometric parameters in various chronic diseases. Nearly all participants viewed the combined video and counseling services as the preferred method to video alone, and with appropriate education toward telehealth utilization they demonstrated high usability of the technology platform. In the aggregate, codesigns and teleassistance are novel examples of the implementation methods older adult patients require to overcome common telehealth barriers such as frailty, cognitive decline, and a lack of caregiver support. As we continue to expand telehealth implementation in older adults, within current models of care, there will be situations in which video visits alone cannot sufficiently address the complexity of care required. These connections harness five core competencies important for digital technologies when used for older adult care: (1) identification (entry point in to care); (2) education (benefits and risks of services); (3) engagement (patient empowerment for self-care); (4) service delivery (usable information to inform care and decisions); and (5) remote monitoring (determine the health of a patient away from a clinic visit). A cohesive ecosystem of information technology and patient participation in remote monitoring such as this aims to identify the right patients for the right services at the right time.

While the use of telemedicine in the elderly may not be the right fit for every patient, pre-visit considerations for enrollment in a telemedicine model should include the following: comfort or prior use with current technology, whether there is existing home support for technology during the televisit such as availability of nursing or family members, development of clear instructions for optimizing the audio-visual experience-including nuances such as testing that speakers are functional and that a hearing aid or other device is both adequately battery-powered where appropriate, and will not cause interference with audio input. Many older adults are already incorporating technology for daily use such as smart home technology with voice assistance in addition to wearable fitness monitors to measure activity, smart scales, home blood pressure, oxygen saturation and sleep monitors, in addition to medication reminder alerts on their personal devices. There has also been an emergence of senior tailored technology such as gait assessment tools for fall risk alerts and connected hearing aids which can provide clinician feedback [6]. Increasing utilization by providers was further supported by the decision to expand reimbursement for remote patient monitoring by the Centers for Medicare & Medicaid Services in 2019.

With this surge of tech use, it is helpful to have a plan for common technical pitfalls, which may be increasingly important for telemonitoring strategies. Older patients may not have the experience with technology to deal with device troubleshooting issues. Some of these include sensor failure and battery life for wearables, network connectivity or privacy failure. Monitoring program integration will also include clinical decision support issues related to translating collected data in appropriate algorithms into a concise recommendation for both patients and providers, and communication of sensor data and recommendations in a usable, easily interpreted form. Other practical considerations are associated with frequency of assessment of captured data and need for follow up to help balance the need for risk assessment over time in addition to avoiding dreaded "data overload" seen with continuous data sets such as heart rhythm and intracardiac pressures [6]. Some of this may need to be tailored to the patient's current clinical status, individual health literacy, and ability to facilitate both in person and/or real time telemedicine follow ups as needed.

8.2   Disabilities

Cardiovascular virtual care management also requires proactive processes to address visual, auditory, cognitive and physical impairments. Despite video format becoming more predominant in modern society's communication, accessibility for disabled patients among digital platforms remains limited. Currently the technical standards for telemedicine as it relates to patients with disabilities are voluntary. Certain disabilities will require development of custom features and technology in addition to patient information tools targeted for disability accommodations. The Americans with Disabilities Act (ADA) mostly protects patients with disabilities in physical spaces as it was developed earlier than the emergence of broad use of the virtual space for health care delivery. This unfortunate truth may be a source of poor consequences for patients with certain disabilities, and will need to continue to be a topic of further development as digital platforms become further tailored for medical care in order to promote inclusivity in telemedicine and to honor patients' civil rights to equal access to healthcare. The COVID-19 pandemic did force some of these virtual spaces and produced data to suggest that telemedicine in patients with disabilities lowered cost of care and need for paid personal assistance, lowered transportation cost, decreased exposure to communicable diseases and improved medication reconciliation [7]. In the following segment we will review some specific considerations.

Slight visual disturbances, color blindness, photosensitivity, peripheral vision loss and total blindness are some examples of the wide variety of visual impairments experienced by older patients. In developing virtual visit environments, providers and patients should be made aware of platform accessibility features including screen magnification, resizing of images and text, audio description aides, text alternatives for images, consistent navigation mechanisms, color contrast settings, and full keyboard navigation. It is helpful to understand if the platform in use is compatible with assistive devices such as Braille keyboards and screen readers [6]. It is also important to understand how stored medical information is shared to patients via patient portals and the methods by which patients and caregivers can access their health information and communicate with providers in less traditional ways.

An estimated 466 million people worldwide have disabling hearing loss [8]. Auditory disabilities may also be addressed in virtual care. For those patients with mild auditory dysfunction, ensuring there is no background noise during the visit and confirming the patient is not getting feedback from assistive devices such as their hearing aids may suffice to improve the patient experience. For more severe auditory issues or total deafness, captions, transcripts of conversation, or inclusion of ASL interpreters for the video visit may assist in a more comfortable experience. It is also helpful to be aware of and instruct the patient about the volume controls and confirm the media is working for them prior to conducting the medical portion of the visit.

Cognitive disabilities pose unique challenges to communication even in live environments, and can range broadly to include mild speech impediments, post-concussive symptoms, neurobehavioral and intellectual disabilities, mental health disorders, dementia and post stroke symptomatology more prevalent in elderly populations. In addition to vision and hearing issues as discussed above, motor skills, expressive and receptive communication issues, and neurologic symptoms whether transient or permanent can affect the success of virtual visits in this population. Very elderly patients over 85 year of age make up 17% of all stroke patients [9], and have higher disability, higher risk-adjusted mortality, and are less likely to be discharged to their original place of residence. A recent study evaluated the impact of confinement in the setting of the COVID-19 pandemic on the health and well-being of community-dwelling older adults (mean age 73.34) with mild cognitive impairment or mild dementia, utilizing a television-based and telephone-based assistive integrated technology. While they found no difference in the physical and mental health and well-being of this vulnerable population, they found participants living alone reported greater negative feelings and more sleeping problems, and the technology allowed for cognitive stimulation by way of engagement in memory games in addition to a useful tool for dissemination of patient-centered information, reinforcing the importance of gauging patients' tech and health literacy prior to utilization of digital health delivery methods [10]. Determining whether a patient is a good candidate for a virtual visit, whether additional devices are necessary for success and if the presence of a caregiver is recommended for some or all of the encounter is an important early step. For example, in patients with speech disabilities, accessibility aides to consider include voice synthesizers and text to speech generators which should be explored prior to conducting your first visit [6]. Note, some platforms allow for caregivers to be included remotely if they are not physically with the patient at the time of the encounter. It is important that providers obtain patient consent for including caregivers or family members- though this is often considered implied—much like when a patient brings their family member for an in person visit. If there are multiple people included in the virtual visit, it is helpful to start with focused introductions of the role they play in the patient's life and medical care.

Patients with physical impairments, challenges with transport, need for gait assistance or supervision and chronic pain may benefit from virtual care options. Often requiring coordination for transport services depending on degree of disability, virtual visits when appropriate can be more cost effective, take less time to complete, and convenient for patients and caregivers. They also provide a unique opportunity to understand the home environment which can be explored further in a video visit and is instrumental to ensure the physically disabled are adequately equipped and risk stratified to avoid falls and/or other comorbidity. Additionally virtual platforms should have large consistent navigation controls to assist in usability for those patients who may experience fine motor movement disorders.

8.3 Palliative Care

While telemedicine modalities have been increasingly incorporated in the field of palliative care due to its multidisciplinary nature, its utilization was greatly accelerated by the need for social distancing during the COVID-19 pandemic. There is certainly a role for telemedicine in assisting patients attain their end of life goals with dignity. In Calton et al.'s recent review of telemedicine for palliative care in the time of COVID-19, they discuss high rates (greater than 97%) of comfort in having "sensitive and emotional conversations by video" from an unpublished manuscript conducted at UCSF assessing patient and caregiver satisfaction rates of 35 palliative care patients who had at least one palliative care visit by telemedicine. As patients with complex cardiovascular disease progress, telemedicine visits may offer an appropriate arena for care coordination and a space for often difficult conversations. Some tips recommended by the author for success with telemedicine particularly with sensitive topics include utilizing patient portals to send out a saved set of instructions and expectations for the visit (may use "dot phrases or macros" as allowed by EMR), channel resources to assign a family member or caregiver as a "technical liaison" one to two days prior to the visit to do a test run and troubleshoot technological issues, and remembering to still have personal moments. While virtual visits tend to be shorter and more efficient in terms of time compared to in-person visits, it is recommended to use the time to personalize the experience: acknowledge the barriers of technology, thank patients for their participation in these kinds of visits, and check in with patients about fears, concerns, and personal effects.

8.4 Language Barriers

Language barriers impact most facets of health care, including access, patient-clinician communication, quality of care, and patient safety. Nearly a quarter of the US population speaks a language other than English at home, and 25.6 million Americans (8%) have limited English proficiency [11]. Formal pathways for the integration of interpreter services utilization for telemedicine visits are essential to ensure equitable care for patients who speak English as a second language (Fig. 8.1). Patient education regarding the import of interpreter service utilization is also necessary as many tend to defer to family members for interpreter services. Studies have shown that families randomized to receive video interpretation are more aware of medical diagnoses than those who receive telephonic interpretation and have more consistent interpreter use with no significant differential in hospital charges [13].

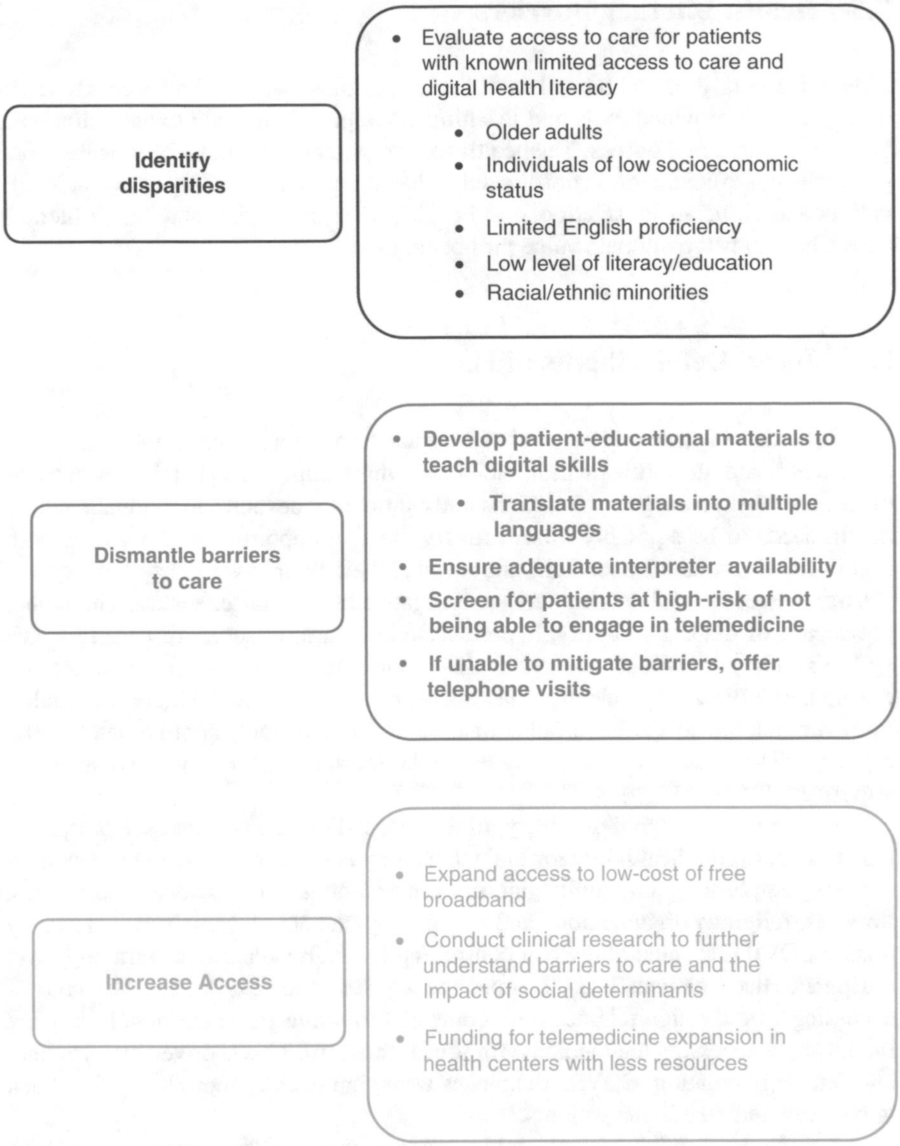

Fig. 8.1 Mechanism to implement equitable access to telemedicine care. Derived from [12]

8.5 Health Literacy Barriers

Elderly patients, those with low health literacy, or those with limited access to technology can be provided tools and teaching to adapt. It is a tactic to help eliminate barriers and increase access. Telehealth has the potential to make healthcare more personalized, efficient, and coordinated; it has the potential to improve efficiency, patient and clinician satisfaction, and health outcomes. Digital and health literacy (See Chap. 9) is the ultimate value proposition.

8.6 Social Determinants of Health

The institution of structural racism has been and remains a fundamental cause of the persistent health disparities within racial and ethnic minorities [14]. It concentrates power amongst privileged populations and continually devalues individual's whose health needs to be equitably improved. By limiting opportunities for social, economic and financial advancement, the racial and ethnic minorities experience reciprocity between social determinants and negative health consequences. The higher prevalence of diabetes, obesity, hypertension and cardiovascular disease in Black and Hispanic populations, has led to disproportionately poorer clinical outcomes during the COVID-19 pandemic. Black Americans experience the highest mortality rates attributable to cardiovascular disease and stroke with approximately 30% higher CVD mortality and 45% higher stroke mortality than non-Hispanic White Americans [15].

Overcoming the digital divide requires increased broadband access, smartphone penetration, digital health literacy and technology education. Rural and urban areas can also emphasize community internet access points such as local pharmacies, libraries, religious organizations and community centers. A New York City study during COVID revealed that when controlling for individual and community-level attributes, Black patients had 0.6 times the adjusted odds (95% CI: 0.58–0.63) of accessing care through telemedicine compared to white patients, though they are increasingly accessing telemedicine for urgent care [16]. This is driven by a younger and female population. COVID diagnoses were significantly more likely for Black versus white telemedicine patients.

A new study found that Black and Hispanic Americans experience a "racial tech gap" and in urban areas, these communities are 10 years behinds the white communities. As of 2019, approximately 10% of adults in the U.S. reported no Internet use, which was largely influenced by Black race, Hispanic ethnicity, older age (>65), and low socioeconomic status [17]. The racial tech gap can be narrowed through community outreach, dismantling barriers to care and health promotion education. Proactive efforts to ensure equity in the current wide-scale implementation of telemedicine need to acknowledge and address disparities in healthcare access for disenfranchised populations with limited digital literacy or access to technology, such as rural residents, racial and ethnic minorities, the elderly, individuals of low socioeconomic status or limited English proficiency. Digital inequity may start as early as middle school and can set individuals back in the digital generation. Lack of access to hardware and broadband data, poor digital literacy and limited English proficiency may foster bias, decrease telehealth access, exacerbate inequities in delivery of care and worsen clinical outcomes in marginalized patients with cardiovascular disease [12].

The etiology of disparate telemedicine uptake are complex and reflect individual, community and structural factors. While digital literacy and hesitancy to adopt new ways of patient-provider interactions have both been shown to widen the digital divide for elderly patients [18], socioeconomic status may serve as a more significant driver for reduced access to health technology, reduced engagement telemedicine, and poor adoption of digital health among Non-Hispanic Black and Hispanic patients. Funding local digital navigators, offering and covering audio-only televisits, providing sustainable discounts for broadband will aid in limiting the digital divide. Many advocacy groups are pushing the government in the US to provide universal broadband access as a basic utility. It will hopefully be expanded to allow healthcare, education and other necessary industries to reach vulnerable populations, however it may also fall on the healthcare industry to offer connected care in clinically vulnerable populations at strategic times (i.e. post hospital discharge, during cardiac rehabilitation, and while titrating medications), or for longitudinal care. Companies need to emphasize that telemedicine platforms should be available in multiple languages at the front end to maximize user experience.

References

1. Narasimha S, Madathil KC, Agnisarman S, Rogers H, Welch B, Ashok A, et al. Designing telemedicine systems for geriatric patients: a review of the usability studies. Telemed J E Health. 2017;23(6):459–72.
2. Calton B, Abedini N, Fratkin M. Telemedicine in the time of coronavirus. J Pain Symptom Manag. 2020;60(1):e12–4.
3. Sarfo FS, Ulasavets U, Opare-Sem OK, Ovbiagele B. Tele-rehabilitation after stroke: an updated systematic review of the literature. J Stroke Cerebrovasc Dis. 2018;27(9):2306–18.
4. Zhu Y, Gu X, Xu C. Effectiveness of telemedicine systems for adults with heart failure: a meta-analysis of randomized controlled trials. Heart Fail Rev. 2020;25(2):231–43.
5. De Cola MC, Maresca G, D'Aleo G, Carnazza L, Giliberto S, Maggio MG, et al. Teleassistance for frail elderly people: a usability and customer satisfaction study. Geriatr Nurs. 2020;41(4):463–7.
6. BoIA. Rising to meet the telehealth accessibility challenge in the time of COVID-19. 2020. https://www.boia.org/blog/rising-to-meet-the-telehealth-accessibility-challenge-in-the-time-of-covid-19
7. Annaswamy TM, Verduzco-Gutierrez M, Frieden L. Telemedicine barriers and challenges for persons with disabilities: COVID-19 and beyond. Disabil Health J. 2020;13(4):100973.
8. World Health Organization. Deafness and hearing loss: key facts. 2020. http://www.who.int/news-room/fact-sheets/detail/deafness-and-hearing-loss.

9. Benjamin EJ, Virani SS, Callaway CW, Chamberlain AM, Chang AR, Cheng S, et al. Heart disease and stroke statistics—2018 update: a report from the American Heart Association. Circulation. 2018;137(12):e67–e492.

10. Goodman-Casanova JM, Dura-Perez E, Guzman-Parra J, Cuesta-Vargas A, Mayoral-Cleries F. Telehealth home support during COVID-19 confinement for community-dwelling older adults with mild cognitive impairment or mild dementia: survey study. J Med Internet Res. 2020;22(5):e19434. https://doi.org/10.2196/19434. PMID: 32401215; PMCID: PMC7247465

11. Flores G. Language barriers and hospitalized children: are we overlooking the most important risk factor for adverse events? JAMA Pediatr. 2020;174(12):e203238. https://doi.org/10.1001/jamapediatrics.2020.3238.

12. Nouri S, Khoong EC, Lyles CR, Karliner L. Addressing equity in telemedicine for chronic disease management during the COVID-19 pandemic. NEJM Catal Innov Care Deliv. 2020; https://doi.org/10.1056/CAT.20.0123. https://doi.org/10.1056/CAT.20.0123

13. Jacobs EA, Vela M. Reducing language barriers in health care: is technology the answer? JAMA Pediatr. 2015;169(12):1092–3. https://doi.org/10.1001/jamapediatrics.2015.3022.

14. Churchwell K, Elkind MS, Benjamin RM, Carson AP, Chang EK, Lawrence W, American Heart Association, et al. Call to action: structural racism as a fundamental driver of health disparities: a presidential advisory from the American Heart Association. Circulation. 2020;142(24):e454–68.

15. Centers for Disease Control and Prevention (CDC). About underlying cause of death, 1999–2018. 2020. https://wonder.cdc.gov/ucd-icd10.html. Accessed 13 Aug 2020.

16. Chunara R, Zhao Y, Chen J, Lawrence K, Testa PA, Nov O, Mann DM. Telemedicine and healthcare disparities: a cohort study in a large healthcare system in New York City during COVID-19. J Am Med Inform Assoc. 2021;28(1):33–41. https://doi.org/10.1093/jamia/ocaa217. PMID: 32866264; PMCID: PMC7499631

17. Walia A, & Ravindran S. America's racial gap & big tech's closing window. 2020. https://www.dbresearch.com/PROD/RPS_EN-PROD/America%27s_Racial_Gap_%26_Big_Tech%27s_Closing_Window/RPS_EN_DOC_VIEW.calias?rwnode=PROD0000000000464258&ProdCollection=PROD0000000000511664

18. Levy H, Janke AT, Langa KM. Health literacy and the digital divide among older Americans. J Gen Intern Med. 2015;30(3):284–9. https://doi.org/10.1007/s11606-014-3069-5

Chapter 9
Education in Virtual Care Delivery: Clinician Education and Digital Health Literacy

Kevin Fickenscher and Jaclyn A. Pagliaro

When layered together, the sharing and integration of information to create knowledge is radically altering our traditional approach to the production of all goods and services. Individuals are now empowered to bypass traditional avenues and methods of resource access (e.g. transportation, housing). Even the knowledge traditionally held by certain professional categories or trades (e.g. lawyers, architects—and, yes, even physicians) is now open, accessible and free. Digital technologies and capabilities have already begun to dramatically alter our approach toward solving traditional problems by enabling new applications of innovation and creativity in specific domains. For the healthcare community—the information revolution is creating a profound reconsideration of the who, what, where, when and how of the entire health care delivery model.

Information and knowledge sharing are the underlying forces for driving transformative change in healthcare. This phenomenon coupled with the diversification of the workforce, emerging technologies and the march towards alternative payment systems designed to foster value-based care delivery, are precipitating new models of care delivery throughout the world.

Cardiology is not isolated from the many changes sweeping the healthcare landscape. In fact, the reliance of the specialty on the digitization of information to support accurate diagnostic and treatment approaches has only accelerated in recent years. What started as a mere computerized analysis of the EKG in the formative years of the information revolution has turned into augmented intelligence during all manner of cardiovascular procedures. The end result is an increased need for

K. Fickenscher (✉)
Northeastern University Bouve College of Health Sciences, Boston, MA, USA

CREO Strategic Solutions, Kittery, ME, USA
e-mail: drkevin@creostrategicsolutions.com

J. A. Pagliaro
Corrigan Minehan Heart Center, Massachusetts General Hospital, Boston, MA, USA

© Springer Nature Switzerland AG 2021   111
A. B. Bhatt (ed.), *Healthcare Information Technology for Cardiovascular Medicine*, Health Informatics, https://doi.org/10.1007/978-3-030-81030-6_9

Structure	Process	Outcomes
The implementation of an academic training program focused on existing clinicians providing telehealth care	A core curriculum needs to be defined that applicable to practicing clinicians focused on continuing ed	The efficiency, utilization, efficacy and clinical outcome measures provide the framework for effectiveness of training

Fig. 9.1 Steps for successful development and implementation of telemedicine education

effective education regarding the capabilities and trends of cardiovascular digital transformation.

Education regarding cardiovascular digital transformation is necessary for several industries. It is important for the general cardiologist to first understand what health IT looks like today, which areas are most promising for forward progress in cardiology and how to take advantage of these technologies. Health system executives are assessing the opportunities to change the infrastructure of cardiovascular care delivery. Nonprofits and private equity are actively seeking out medical expertise and evaluation of which technologies will improve healthcare through addressing social determinants of health centered around access. Broadly available education also allows entrepreneurs in digital health to identify where the challenges lie in incorporating IT and engaging providers in adoption which has been a long-standing challenge for the digital health world (Fig. 9.1).

9.1 A Brief Exploration of the Transformative Forces Affecting the Delivery of Healthcare

The pace of change we are witnessing in health care requires a reassessment of our approach toward the training of medical and health sciences clinical providers. These changes will only accelerate in the coming decades as the Digital and Information Revolutions continue to evolve. What are the major factors causing the revolution in health care?

9.1.1 Economic Globalization

Every nation in every region of the world is seemingly interconnected as a result of technology. Witnessing the recent global pandemic that was not sequestered in one place but spread across the entire world, caused economic as well as care delivery ripples. Economic globalization by its very nature, triggers an unremitting reexamination of cost structures related to the production of all goods and services across multiple industries. Healthcare is not immune to these changes. As the use of virtual care technologies expand, some authorities are predicting the "internationalization" of health care delivery much like we have seen in areas of the economy [1, 2].

9.1.2 Cost of Health Care

The strain on the federal budget from Medicare/Medicaid (26%) and Social Security (24%) [3] alone is resulting in political backlash from other sectors requiring federal or state government support. With the recent debt incurred by the COVID-19 pandemic, these pressures on local, state and federal government will only increase. It is an increasingly recognized imperative among the political establishment that the escalation of healthcare costs must be reined in and managed more effectively.

As technologies such as Bluetooth enabled devices, ambient pressure monitors and wearables are now able to track the weight, vitals and respiratory fluctuations continuously in patients allowing for much earlier diagnostic interventions to prevent high cost care delivery in emergency rooms and hospitalizations. Appropriately deployed technology can alter this pattern by using various technology-related resources that create increased efficiency, enhanced effectiveness, improved quality and better outcomes.

9.1.3 Societal and Provider Demographics

Societal demographics are shifting across the world. Over the last century, the average life expectancy for individuals has increased dramatically. The United States has not been immune to this trend. According to the U.S. Census Bureau, the country is "aging". Over the period between 2012 and 2050, the number of people aged 65 will have grown from approximately 43 million to nearly 84 million individuals, with the Boomer generation representing the bulk of that growth [4].

9.1.4 Shifting Reimbursement Models

For much of the last century, healthcare in the U.S. has been based on a fee-for-service (FFS) payment model. Although the exact trajectory is not yet clear, the movement in a new direction toward value-based payment models in care delivery seems imminent. Such a shift will inevitably result in a change of how groups of physicians and hospitals operate with the result that quality, efficiency, and effectiveness outcomes likely to dominate the models for care delivery.

9.1.5 Social Determinants of Health

There is an increased recognition that the social determinants of health (SDOH), are major factors in predicting outcomes and quality of care. The CDC recommends focusing on five key areas across the SDOH continuum, including: (1) economic stability, (2) education, (3) social and community context, (4) health and health care; and, (5) neighborhood and built environment. These key considerations represent the major contributing factors related to the overall health of individuals and the community as well as the eventual cost of care. In addition, it is now widely recognized that a sixth dimension must also be considered as a key element for addressing social determinants—addressing cultural competencies and health disparities [5, 6]. The move toward values-based payment and delivery models coupled with a solid foundation integration of the six major social determinants is another transformation force altering the future of care delivery.

9.1.6 Rapidity of Technology Advancement

Biotechnology, genomics, nanomedicine, robotics and changes in pharmaceutical development are a few examples of many breakthroughs occurring in healthcare. The pace of change and its direct impact on the delivery of care is quickening. The capability of medical devices, drugs and delivery mechanisms and their impact on where and how care is delivered is far greater today than at any point in human history, and their future impact will be highly significant.

One area of technology use that is now at the forefront is the application of telehealth services. Interest in the use of virtual care delivery models was slowly increasing until the global pandemic when there was a precipitous increase in interest us the use of telehealth and virtual visit services.

9.1.7 Summary of Driving Forces

All these forces are driving a disintermediation of the entire care delivery process and must be addressed by healthcare organizations. While the list is not exhaustive, these forces are requiring the industry to rapidly adopt improvements in its value proposition through transformation. To assure that the results of the healthcare enterprise are "safe, effective, efficient, timely, patient-centered, and equitable" [7] as well as beneficial. Meeting these challenges requires leadership at all levels and a basic reconfiguration of the care delivery model. Virtual services will no doubt be a central component as care delivery models are redesigned over the coming decade.

9.2 Education and Training: Requirements for Virtual Care Delivery

One of the major impediments to expanding virtual care delivery is insufficient formal training for clinicians related to the application, use and benefits of utilizing these new and evolving virtual technologies. Healthcare providers across all specialties, will require training in telemedicine skills to meet the demands of digitally empowered patients as well as to deliver care in the new digital age of medicine.

There is an immediate need to define the requirements of a core curriculum in telemedicine training. The four main components will include continuous remote monitoring, individually relevant predictive algorithms, asynchronous patient data and virtual video visits, which form the foundation for sustainable telemedicine care. Over time, specialties such as cardiology, which are remarkably data driven, will witness even more changes through the application of machine learning and artificial intelligence.

9.2.1   What Training Will Virtualist Care Clinicians Require?

Virtual clinicians and care providers will not typically be co-located with patients and other members of the health care team. Therefore, their training must emphasize specific competencies in leading and participating in interdisciplinary teams distributed across multiple workspaces and environments. Training in informatics, analytics and population health will prepare virtual providers to separate signals from noise in large dynamic sets of patient data, allowing decisive action without the absolute requirement of the traditional physical examination. Although formal training in the above domains will become more prevalent as all medical specialties and health care fields adapt to the demands of the information age, deeper competencies in these fields will differentiate the virtual health clinicians from care providers with a baseline or generalist level of virtual skills training (Table 9.1).

9.2.2   Elements of Virtual Health Care Training:
             The Core Curriculum

The core curriculum for virtual care delivery has been established and revised by several national organizations. Each emphasizes providing clinicians the knowledge required to successfully deliver basic virtual care. Specialized tracks and advanced training in the nuances of care delivery, devices and data analysis will evolve over time.

American Medical Association (AMA) adopted the policy in 2016 during its Annual Meeting to encourage the adoption of telemedicine training for medical students and residents. While the policy specifically encouraged undergraduate and graduate medical education accreditation bodies to include core competencies for telemedicine in their programs, no such formal guidelines have been forthcoming to date. Furthermore, the AMA recommendations were restricted to the concept of telemedicine and did not include consideration of telemonitoring and telecare, two important elements of the proposed telehealth educational framework.

Table 9.1 Four critical principles for developing and deploying a virtual health training program

1. Interdisciplinary/ Interprofessional/Team-based care is an essential modality in a virtual environment.	In a value-based approach to health care delivery, the importance of a fully functional and integrated team approach becomes an essential component of the care provider team. The essentials of team development, inter-professional communications and use of virtual capabilities in such environments must be a focus for the training of health care virtualists.
2. Clinically augmented intelligence is a capability, not a replacement.	The intent of virtual health care training is not to replace clinicians but to arm them with the tools and technologies that can clearly augment their capabilities in providing quality, cost-effective care. Therefore, how virtual tools are effectively integrated with face-to-face care delivery is an important element in the education of virtual health care clinicians.
3. Telemedicine skills apply across the continuum of health professionals	In adopting virtual care models, it is important for all care delivery professionals to understand how, when, where and what virtual tools should be used in augmenting the care of the team. Therefore, training is not restricted to just a few clinicians but is encouraged for all members of the health care team.
4. Inter-institutional collaboration will accelerate the ability of higher education to respond to the shifting care delivery environment.	A comprehensive approach is required if clinicians are to be provided the breadth of training required to shift from traditional face-to-face models of care delivery toward the integration of virtual health models. Many residency programs are hospital-based in non-academic settings or in academic settings without the requisite talents in all the proposed domains. In such an environment, collaboration among the health science training programs of the nation should be considered a mainstay of implementation.

In the absence of clear accreditation requirements by the medical education community, the American Telemedicine Association adopted an Accreditation Program for Online Patient Consultations in 2015. The focus of the accreditation requirements; however, is on the more operational aspects of telemedicine including patient safety, transparency of operations and adherence to all relevant laws and regulations. The academic training requirements for clinicians providing such services are not a component of the overall accreditation program.

What if I miss something? The fortunate aspect of virtual visits is that follow up is always possible in some format. Sequential virtual visits, in-person visits, vital signs from home, ordering or reviewing labs and imaging, and leaning on local care providers are all mechanisms to ensure that a virtual visit never stands alone as a patient evaluation tool if there is clinical uncertainty (Table 9.2).

Digital assessment tools will be essential in the future of at-home assessment. Physical metrics such as frailty assessments can be performed in patients' homes using technology or over video and may significantly influence prognosis. Moving

Table 9.2 Conducting a virtual physical exam

Video physical exam
General: Appearance, distress, home environment, visual medication reconciliation
HEENT: Oropharynx, extraocular movements, sclera
Chest: Respiratory rate, retractions, cough
Cardiac: JVP, radial pulse
Abdomen: Visual inspection, tenderness to palpitation
Extremities: Cyanosis, clubbing, edema
Neuro: AAOx3, cranial nerve exam, gross motor, drawing for fine motor
Psych: Behavior, speech, mood, affect, family dynamics

quickly to validate virtual, at-home frailty assessment is another example of existing will enable us to map a patient's specific healthcare needs.

Preparing for Successful Provider and Patient Experience in a Virtual Visit

1. Create a comfortable environment and the right ambiance while avoiding provider frustration with the connection. Pre-visit, educate clinicians regarding optimal lighting (avoiding backlight, using an extra light source), and strong connection (ensure Wi-Fi connection as well as network access). Have a colleague review their workspace virtually to notice what scene the background creates. As the visit commences, educate clinicians to ask the patient if they can see and hear them clearly before beginning. Have at-the-elbow tech support ready when needed as well as a back-up stand-alone platform for phone or video should the technology become frustrating for either party.

2. Make sure patients can connect and arrive with ease. A unique feature of virtual visits is logging in from the comfort of home. Avoiding discontent with the log-on process optimizes this advantage. Practices with medical assistants should train them as part of the workflow to call patients for test visits in advance. It is the clinician's responsibility to educate the medical assistant as to what information they may also want in advance of the appointment that a medical assistant could obtain (i.e., medication reconciliation, social and family history review, chief complaint or concern for the visit, refill requests). Unique accommodations should be noted, including interpreter services, caregiver inclusion, and audiovisual or learning impairment. At the same time, medical assistants should ask patients if they have BP monitors, a scale and other tools to enhance their virtual experience. If so, patients will be asked to upload the data prior to their telehealth visit.

9.3 Educating the Virtual Educator

Virtual education requires clinicians to alter the mechanism by which they teach. A virtual educator, whether teaching a patient and their family or fellow clinicians or trainees needs to serve as designer, director, animator, writer, content expert, engagement expert and communicator (Table 9.3). These are skill sets that one must now adopt in addition to clinical acumen and patient rapport. When taught correctly however, the effect of a good virtual educator is exponential on patient engagement, self-advocacy and compliance. Teaching these skills internally in a clinical practice, telemedicine company or academic medical institution is more challenging than outsourcing skill advancement to the many presentation skill building services available globally. For individuals who have a penchant for large volume virtual clinical practice, we strongly recommend bolstering their bedside manner with formal training in screen side manner as well.

When engaging with individual patients, or patients and families or caregivers, professional set-up, adequate lighting, confirming clear audio and video are the baseline goals as reviewed. Increasing engagement is the next goal with visual diagrams for education, screen sharing of cardiac imaging with basic live annotation to decode complex echocardiography or MRI, and whiteboard use to write out the key action items for the visit can engage patients with auditory, visual and written cues to adapt to all learning styles.

In the setting of group virtual visits, or virtual education of colleagues, additional engagement tools including audience polling, use of breakout rooms, live annotations and sketching, sticky notes for collaboration and repeated use of a concise messaging slide to repeat key goals or educational points. Depending on the situation, including Ted-style storytelling to draw in the audience can also be an effective tool for virtual engagement. Lastly, in challenging virtual patient group interactions or clinical settings, audience synchronization (i.e., simulating a room with participants sitting around a table) and blending physical and virtual interaction (i.e., "passing a ball" to the next speaker) can be useful tools for group engagement.

9.4 Educating the Patient: Digital Health Literacy

Digital health literacy can be defined as a set of skills, knowledge, and attitudes that a person needs to engage with, comprehend and apply health information to their own care. Improving digital health literacy can increase engagement with and the efficacy of virtual and telehealth-based preventive, chronic disease management and acute care in an informed manner. While many adults globally own smartphones, having access to a video- and data-enabled device does not guarantee having the digital skills to use a specific video application to conduct a visit [8]. Lack of broadband access may also be a barrier to video visits, as broadband often facilitates better video quality and does not usually come with a monthly cap on data as seen

Table 9.3 Minimum baseline for training clinicians as generalists in virtual care delivery

Health informatics (HI)	Information engineering for managing and using patient care information. According to HIMSS, the Healthcare Information and Management Systems Society, HI promotes the understanding, integration and application of information technology in the health care setting to ensure adequate and qualified support of clinician objectives and industry best practices.
Artificial intelligence/machine Learning	Systems used in artificial intelligence and machine learning are expanding and moving in new directions as the technology continues to evolve. As a result, the area is dynamic and requires both an understanding of current capabilities, directions of research and possible derivative capabilities that could evolve from integration of multiple, independent data sets.
Social media	Integrating social media and health care data is required to more effectively track and intervene in the consumer health care experience and identify population health trends on a real-time rather than retrospective basis.
Immersive media	Health care is experiencing technological disruption and the adoption of immersive media tools as a part of the transformational change in care delivery. Immersive media—including virtual reality and augmented reality—are broadening how people learn and heal and how we can facilitate and accelerate their behavioral changes. The use of immersive media environments holds the potential for accelerating behavioral change in patients by supporting education on all aspects of medical, health and/or social considerations that play a role in the health of individuals.
Psychology of virtual Communications	Many industries have benefitted from recent advancements in the use of video communication technologies. These new capabilities have allowed individuals the opportunity to express their perspectives, ideas and concerns in ways that may not present in as forthcoming a manner as direct, in-person communications. However, the health care field is only at the nascent stage of using these new tools. As face-to-face communication lessens and as health care adopts more virtual communications, the need for training in the best approaches to avoid the potential for miscommunication from the use of texts, chats, e-mails and other forms becomes apparent. Virtual care providers must learn the psychology of these virtual communications tools and how they can affect the patient-clinician interface.
Inter-professional and virtual team management	Many organizations across multiple industries have learned that it is important to focus on effective team management in virtual environments. Issues such as process and task clarification, establishing a communication charter, use of communication technologies and shared language and nomenclature are but a few of the examples of areas where cross-team training is required. Handoffs within, across and beyond the team are particularly important for virtual care providers since these handoffs can have a direct impact on the care of the individual patient.
Remote care delivery and operational requirements for supporting virtual care delivery	This area of is quite dynamic with new technologies emerging at an increasingly rapid pace. Students will learn the best approaches for effective analysis of the latest research in the rapidly evolving virtual remote care delivery space, a prime consideration in this section.

(continued)

Table 9.3 (continued)

Technical Innovations and trends	It is very clear that health care's technical evolution has often been far ahead of the practical application of its tools and technologies. Virtual health care providers must become more expert in evaluating such technologies to assist their organizations in determining the appropriateness of deployment.
Frameworks for effective technology assessment	As virtual technologies move into mainstream health care, virtual care providers will be called upon to assist their organizations in assessing technologies to improve efficiency, access and quality of health care, as well as how to deploy such tools in support of care delivery. The interests of such clinicians will naturally shift towards evidence-based medicine, comparative effectiveness research and health technology assessment (HTA) tools. Therefore, virtual care providers must be adequately trained in the systematic approach to evidence, relevant outcomes in support of care delivery, and other dimensions of technology and the frameworks used for supporting such assessments.
Legal, regulatory, privacy and security requirements	As the field evolves, understanding the changing dynamics of the oversight requirements and overarching strategic confidentiality of information derived through virtual systems must be a core area of understanding

with cell phone plans. Even when accessible, many patient-facing web pages, medical health records accessible through online portals and mobile health applications are not optimized for patients with low digital health literacy [9]. Age, educational attainment, digital literacy and health literacy independently, health status, trust in healthcare and digital information, their motivation for seeking information, accommodations for limitations, and ability to co-engage with family members or support persons are among the key factors which influence digital health literacy and must be addressed in the infrastructure of digital health tools and sites during their design [10]. Approximately 25% of Americans do not have the digital literacy skills or access to the technology required to engage in video visits.

9.4.1 Health Literacy

Health literacy is the degree to which individuals are able to access and process basic health information and services and are thereby able to participate in health-related decisions. Limited health literacy is highly prevalent worldwide and is strongly associated with patient morbidity, mortality, healthcare utilization and costs. It has also been associated with limited knowledge of health conditions and medications, poorer overall health status, higher healthcare costs, and increased likelihood of rehospitalization and mortality. Online medical education, technical instructions, and any self-scheduling mechanisms when offered only in English, presents a significant barrier to care. In cardiovascular disease, health literacy is an invisible barrier to healthcare delivery that has profound costs for individual and public health. It has been associated with poorer outcomes preceding and following coronary events and is associated with

30-day readmission after acute coronary syndromes. In individuals with heart failure, limited health literacy has been associated with 1.3- to 2-fold higher all-cause mortality in hospital and community-based cohorts. Individuals with limited health literacy experience barriers to referral to, engagement with, and participation in cardiac rehabilitation services and thus miss the physiological and non-physiological benefits after coronary events. Multisession telephone-based intervention for individuals with heart failure led to a lower likelihood of hospitalization. A cross-sectional study of 402 patients from 2 racially diverse and geographically distinct public, urban healthcare facilities found that the majority (55%) of individuals with inadequate health literacy were not able to recognize a blood pressure of 160/100 mm Hg as abnormal.

Interventions addressing health literacy in individuals with CVD have focused primarily on medication adherence including reminders, illustrated medication schedules, and even pharmacist assisted medication reconciliation and counseling. Telephone follow up appears promising as well. The addition of video, the ability for a clinician to see how medications are stored, assist with labeling real time, review storage location and incorporate caregivers in the conversation from home, may all prove to address health literacy in a more tangible way.

Chat messaging using smart phones has evolved as a mechanism to provide direct feedback and patient engagement (https://www.ahajournals.org/doi/full/10.1161/CIRCOUTCOMES.119.005805) (Table 9.4).

Individuals with limited health literacy face challenges in accessing and navigating health care, and such obstacles may be exacerbated by family, community, and social factors. Only 12% of US adults have the health literacy skills to navigate its complexity

Table 9.4 Examples of text messages used in the CHAT-DM randomized controlled trial

General information on CHD and DM [1×/wk]
Diabetes is not terrible and there are many things you can do to prevent problems from diabetes, such as monitoring blood glucose, watching your diet, keeping fit, and taking pills regularly.

Glucose monitoring and control [1×/wk]
Afraid of testing blood glucose because it hurts? Try to test on the sides of your fingertips or rotate your fingers, which can help to minimize pain.

Blood pressure control [1×/wk]
Home blood pressure monitoring is highly recommended! You can get an accurate picture of your heart health and understand daily changes in blood pressure, which is helpful for doctors to adjust medications for you.

Medication adherence [1×/wk]
Taking diabetes medications or injecting insulin regularly can help control your blood glucose level. Forgetting to take your medication? Try to set a repeating alarm on your cell phone to remind you to take medication or insulin injection.

Physical activity [1×/wk]
Regular exercise is important for managing diabetes, physical activities such as aerobic exercise and strength training can help you to make your body use insulin better and reduce the risk for heart disease and osteoporosis.

Lifestyle recommendations [1×/wk]
The sugary drink may have an adverse impact on your weight and blood glucose. Try to drink water as it is simply the best choice when you are thirsty.

Fig. 9.2 Components of
digital health literacy

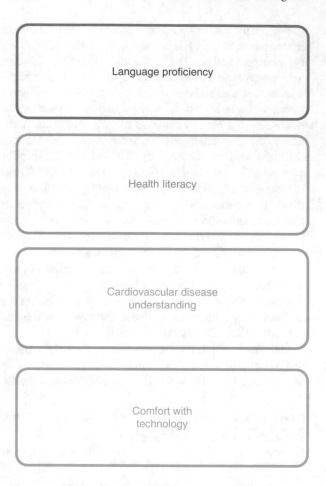

successfully [11]. The AHRQ Universal Precautions Toolkit for Health Literacy is a publicly available document focused on improving quality of care. [12] It identifies the attributes of a health-literate organization and provides guidance for cardiovascular centers. The American Heart Association has also authored a scientific statement [13] on health literacy in cardiovascular disease. In that they suggest strategies that address barriers created by limited health literacy on the management and prevention of cardio-vascular disease which are applicable to practices offering telemedicine and digital tech-nology companies developing platforms or devices for telehealth care alike (Fig. 9.2).

9.5   Summary

New technological capabilities, advances in virtual care delivery, changing societal expectations and a burgeoning demand for basic care services have created a new venue for care delivery outside of traditional face-to-face environments (Table 9.5).

Table 9.5 Future trends in health sciences training

Virtual care training will become embedded in health sciences education	It is highly likely that virtual training will become a core element of the formal education of all medical and health sciences students. As the trend evolves, further specialization in the use of virtual technologies and applications will also evolve.
A continuing education initiative is critical to bring the existing health care workforce up to speed	Certificate programs and specialty updates will no doubt be required for practicing clinicians. Industry-focused training programs on specific tools or platforms may be an insufficient foundation for adequately preparing clinicians to serve as virtual care providers.
Augmented training requirements for specialized virtual medical and health providers	Presently, there are no formal graduate-level training and/or research programs that have been identified in virtual health and care delivery. However, it is anticipated that, within a few short years, such programs will evolve.
Certification of clinicians in virtual health and care delivery will become the norm for individuals involved in virtual care delivery environments	Certification programs within the health care community have been shown to ensure the competence of professionals through a measurement of skills and knowledge with a defined minimum standard.

In addition to educating the clinicians, improving upon health and digital literacy will be essential to patient engagement and improving outcomes with blended care.

Just as physicians and other clinical providers receive a defined grounding in the critical specialties, so they should also be trained in virtualist care capabilities. The purpose of a virtual care training program must be to assist clinicians in understanding common problems and in determining when it is important to seek more traditional as face-to-face care delivery or the assistance of specialists. Further training and skill development are required for all physicians and clinicians who will engage in virtual care delivery so that a baseline of that capability will be a requisite training requirement among all providers. The constant evolution of virtual care paradigms will require modular education offerings ranging from conducting video visits to interpreting patient derived data.

The move toward embracing the virtualist model is an inevitable and essential shift for all medical and clinical professions. The field requires a collaborative approach toward development, implementation and deployment of a rapidly evolving technical landscape. Such collaboration should include universities, associations, industry, health care systems and clinicians as the field of virtual health care continues to evolve and develop.

Case Report

The lead author has served as the driving force for creating a program in virtual care delivery for clinicians involved in providing virtual care delivery. He along with several colleagues in the telehealth and telecare space observed in mid-2015 that the utility of various tele-technology tools was hampered by the fact that front-line clinicians and providers of care who used those tools were inadequately trained. In essence, care providers were often provided very superficial orientations on the technology without any grounding on the utility of the tools or how those tools altered the care delivery process. These observations led to the conclusion that a need existed for a better grounding in telehealth and telecare capabilities. Furthermore, with the pace of change occurring in the industry, a solid grounding in the utility and capability of these tools was becoming increasingly apparent as the technologies continued to expand their delivery capacity.

As a result, in early 2018, the lead author convened a number of thought leaders in the telehealth and telecare industry to discuss the need for and elements of an essential training foundation for clinicians engaged in providing virtual care delivery services. Those formative discussions provided the framework for the ten (10) essential elements of training required for clinicians providing virtual care outlined in this chapter. In addition to the curricular framework, the participants also felt that a program in virtual care delivery should be structured as a *continuing education* initiative rather than as an ancillary degree. Furthermore, the group felt that the capabilities outlined in the core curriculum should be made available to all health care professionals providing clinical support in patient care settings.

Through the remainder of 2018, discussions were held with a number of informatics and health sciences programs across the nation on the feasibility of establishing a "consortium" of schools who would actively support and develop the program. Over time, the complexities of inter-academic collaboration were recognized as an impediment toward a timely implementation of the training program. In the end, Northeastern University based in Boston, Massachusetts stepped forward and indicated a desire to push the initiative forward with the intent that if schools wanted to collaborate in the future, they would welcome their participation. Northeastern University then proceeded to move forward by investing in curricular development and identification of both internal and external resources that could be mobilized to support the proposed curriculum. As of this writing, the Alpha Cohort of participants at Maine Health is completing the program with very positive results and a Beta Cohort of participants from a variety of health care organizations will be initiated in early 2021.

Acknowledgments The author wishes to acknowledge the contributions of the following individuals in assisting efforts to frame the approach toward the development and deployment of effective virtual care training: John Austin, Ph.D. (Fielding Graduate University), Anita Chambers (Odulair, Inc.), Linda Durnell, Ph.D. (Fielding Graduate University), Susan Fenton, Ph.D. (University of Texas Health at Houston), Rosemary Glavan, RN (Independent Consultant), Rebecca Hafner, MD (Zipnosis, Inc.), Gary Hare, Ph.D. (Fielding Graduate University), Joseph Kvedar, MD (Partners Healthcare Center for Connected Health), Joseph Nichols, MD (The MITRE Corporation), Wayne Patterson, Ph.D. (Howard University), Katrina Rogers, Ph.D. (Fielding Graduate University), David Schmitz, MD (University of North Dakota), Donald Warne, MD, Ph.D. (University of North Dakota); and, Joshua Wynne, MD (University of North Dakota).

References

1. Hreinsson J, Woldearegay Y. Internationalization of health care services—networking aspects, Masters thesis, Department of Business Studies, Uppsala Universitet. 2015. http://www.diva-portal.org/smash/get/diva2:786962/FULLTEXT01.pdf

2. Noppen M. The internationalization of health care: the UZ Brussel model for international partnerships. World Hosp Health Serv. 2012;48(4):11–3.
3. Center on Budget and Policy Procedures (CBPP). Policy basics: where do our federal tax dollars go? 2020. https://www.cbpp.org/research/federal-budget/policy-basics-where-do-our-federal-tax-dollars-go
4. Ortman, JM, Velkoff, VA, Hogan H. An aging nation: the older population in the United States. Current population reports. US Bureau of the Census. 2014.
5. Betancourt JR. Cultural competence and medical education: many names, many perspectives, one goal. Acad Med. 2006;81(6):499–501. https://doi.org/10.1097/01.ACM.0000225211.77088.cb.
6. Wagner R, Patow C, Newton R, et al. The overview of the CLER Program: CLER national report of findings 2016. J Grad Med Educ. 2016;8(2 Suppl 1):11–3.
7. Roser M, Ortiz-Ospina E, Ritchie H. Life expectancy. Our world in data. 2013
8. Norman CD, Skinner HA. eHealth literacy: essential skills for consumer health in a networked world. J Med Internet Res. 2006;8(2):e9. https://doi.org/10.2196/jmir.8.2.e9.
9. Sarkar U, Gourley GI, Lyles CR, Tieu L, Clarity C, Newmark L, et al. Usability of commercially available mobile applications for diverse patients. J Gen Intern Med. 2016;31(12):1417–26.
10. Lyles CR, & Sarkar U. Health literacy, vulnerable patients, and health information technology use: where do we go from here?. 2015. https://www.epi.org/publication/health-care-report/
11. Cutilli CC, Bennett IM. Understanding the health literacy of America: results of the National Assessment of Adult Literacy. Orthop Nurs. 2009;28(1):27–34. https://doi.org/10.1097/01.NOR.0000345852.22122.d6
12. AHRQ. Health literacy universal precautions toolkit. 2nd ed. Rockville, MD: Agency for Healthcare Research and Quality; 2020.
13. Magnani JW, Mujahid MS, Aronow HD, Cené CW, Dickson VV, Havranek E, et al. Health literacy and cardiovascular disease: fundamental relevance to primary and secondary prevention: a scientific statement from the American Heart Association. Circulation. 2018;138(2):e48–74.

Chapter 10
Trust in Artificial Intelligence: Clinicians Are Essential

Umang Bhatt and Zohreh Shams

10.1 Introduction

Artificial intelligence (AI) or the use of computational technologies that are inspired by human cognitive functions, is changing the fabric of daily life [1]. From natural language processing for computer readable electronic health records to medical image processing for clinical decision support systems, advances in AI are poised to change the method by which healthcare is delivered [2]. Like other safety and security critical domains, a lack of transparency in AI systems prevents the widespread use of these systems in day-to-day clinical practice. For AI systems to be fully integrated in healthcare practices, they need to be transparent so that the healthcare practitioners can judge when to trust an AI systems' recommendation [3]. In this chapter, we begin with a brief overview of AI, then discuss mechanisms for AI systems to display trustworthiness to external stakeholders and examine the role of the cardiac practitioners in the development and deployment of AI systems.

10.2 Overview of Artificial Intelligence

In the summer of 1956, a handful of scientists convened for the Dartmouth Summer Research Project on Artificial Intelligence. Most agree that this was when the term "artificial intelligence" was coined. To this day, the goal of AI remains the same: to build machines that simulate human intelligence [4, 5]. While simulating human intelligence is an ambitious goal, AI systems in their current form are best suited to augment, not automate humans [6].

U. Bhatt (✉) · Z. Shams
University of Cambridge, Cambridge, UK
e-mail: usb20@cam.ac.uk; zs315@cam.ac.uk

© Springer Nature Switzerland AG 2021   127
A. B. Bhatt (ed.), *Healthcare Information Technology for Cardiovascular Medicine*, Health Informatics, https://doi.org/10.1007/978-3-030-81030-6_10

For healthcare, the utility of AI does not lie in the ability to replace healthcare practitioners, but rather the ability to augment a healthcare practitioners' expertise. The ideal AI system for a healthcare practitioner is one that works alongside the clinician to learn from their behavior and decisions. Several generations of complementary AI systems have been developed and broadly divided into rule-based expert systems, Machine Learning (ML) Driven systems, and hybrid systems that combine expert and ML-Driven systems.

10.2.1   Expert Systems

The role of an expert system is to mirror the reasoning used by an expert when making a decision. The main components are its knowledge base and a reasoning engine, which applies a set of If-Then rules to facts in the knowledge base in order to infer new facts [7, 8].

Example: One of the earliest expert systems, MYCIN [9], was a clinical system developed to identify bacteria causing severe infections, such as meningitis. Based on the diagnosis, MYCIN recommended antibiotics tailored to patients (i.e., adjusted for patients' body weight).

10.2.2   Machine Learning (ML)-Driven Systems

Machine learning applies a hybrid of statistics, computer science and electrical engineering to solve complex problems using large datasets [10]. Unlike expert systems, which rely on experts to provide the desired reasoning, ML-driven systems infer reasoning from data by extracting patterns and identifying interactions from observations and building models that extrapolate to unseen data. This is conducted by identifying interaction patterns among variables. This mechanism does not replace expert reasoning, however, can prove more valuable than user-generated rubric systems. Therefore, in clinical practice, ML can automate decision systems to help physicians make predictions with increased accuracy.

Example: The data used for ML applications in healthcare could include patient information from an electronic health record, medical images, or a clinician's notes. Sometimes labels (or targets) may be provided alongside training data, which indicate the true outcome corresponding to a given input. For example, suppose our training data is a set of medical images, say chest X-rays taken in a hospital. Each chest X-ray is labeled to indicate whether the patient has pneumonia (1) or does not have pneumonia (0). Given these input images and corresponding binary output labels, a ML model can be trained to predict whether a new chest X-ray image contains evidence of pneumonia [11]. The majority of current ML research focuses on creating algorithms to learn an accurate model that performs well on the training data and generalizes to unseen data. The ML-Driven systems in cardiology have followed the same pipeline as explained above and have proven to be able to extract patterns from the data that generalize very well, for example in the diagnosis of heart failure [12].

10.2.3   Hybrid Systems

The most recent generation of healthcare AI systems attempt to rely on both expert knowledge and ML to make recommendations that exploit the known knowledge of practitioners while learning the unknown knowledge emerging from the data.

Example: In [12] a hybrid system for the diagnosis of heart failure is proposed that first formalizes the decision-making of expert clinicians as a set of rules and then it augments that with the rules that come from ML algorithms modeling the cohort of patients with and without heart failure. The hybrid system has proven to be useful, particularly in absence of access to a heart failure specialist. The use of formalized expert knowledge in the format of ontologies (i.e., Gene Ontology [13]) and biological networks is also very common in hybrid approaches [14–17].

10.3   Machine Learning in Healthcare

There are three popular paradigms of machine learning: unsupervised, supervised and reinforcement learning.

In supervised learning, algorithms use a dataset that has been labeled by clinicians, to predict a known outcome. Although supervised learning is ideal for classification and regression problems, it requires a lot of data and is time-consuming because the data has to be labeled by humans. The chest X-ray is a classic example of supervised learning. The ML model is trained on previous chest X-ray data and learns a relationship between the images and the pneumonia labels to then generalize when new chest X-rays are presented.

Unsupervised learning involves training models from data without labels. This is used to parse out insight from the training data itself [18, 19]. Unsupervised learning seeks to identify novel disease mechanisms, genotypes, or phenotypes from patterns in the data, independent of human interpretation. Shah et al. [20] developed an unsupervised learning model to predict the survival of patients with heart failure with preserved ejection fraction (HFpEF). There were 46 distinct variables analyzed which led to three distinct groups. Supervised learning with human input was then utilized to predict the difference in desired outcomes (mortality and hospitalization) among the groups. A significant limitation of unsupervised learning is that the initial cluster pattern must be validated against other cohorts.

Hedman et al. [21] also used machine learning to analyze 32 echocardiograms and 11 clinical and laboratory variables collected from 320 HFpEF outpatients in the Karolinska-Rennes cohort study (56% female, median 78 years; IQR: 71–83) identifying 6 phenogroups.

Reinforcement learning can be crudely seen as a hybrid of supervised and unsupervised learning that aims to maximize the accuracy of algorithms using trial and error. It is well-suited for sequential decision making problems [22, 23]. A full survey of RL in healthcare that ranges from systems that decide treatments for chronic diseases to those that allocate resources within hospitals can be found in [24].

10.3.1   Clinical Data Interpretation Powers AI

Although ML quickly gained traction through the production of large datasets, it has taken more time to be adopted by the healthcare sector [25]. Access to electronic medical records, remote patient data and digital patient-driven data streams can assist in clinical decision making, exploration and discovery when assessed with powerful analytics. As a result of continued collaborations between clinicians and ML researchers, much progress has been made to develop robust methods that adequately consider the variety of data contained in medical data [26, 27]. While these efforts have increased the use of AI in healthcare, the availability of healthcare data is the keystone to unlocking the power of AI in healthcare. Medical data vary per case and are inherently complex. They can include anything from time series data to discrete measures, consisting of signal frequencies, medical images, or text descriptions.

Each type of data requires a different type of preprocessing before being encoded as input features for an ML model. Since clinicians take all of these variables into consideration when deciding diagnosis, prognosis, and treatment, AI systems intended to help clinicians come to these decisions must learn parameters that reflect these considerations. Electronic health records contain rich data that are easily available however, they may be too complex to process [28]. Concurrently, neglecting potentially valuable data can lead to false diagnoses, which can incur unnecessary treatment expenses or cost patient lives. Nevertheless, researcher-clinician collaborations have proved to combat these challenges by informing data collection and processing with clinician expertise. Using a single data structure constructed using the entirety of each patient's chart, Rajkomar et al. [28] were able to predict important clinical outcomes and measure readmission probability.

10.3.1.1   Decision Support

In the healthcare sector, we can augment clinical decision-making by using automated AI systems. Decision support AI systems suggest courses of action but do not implement any actions, therefore, the decision-making power remains with the healthcare practitioner [23]. Augmenting healthcare intelligence takes many forms and clinicians can use AI system outputs to diagnose more efficiently and accurately at a lower cost.

To build a productive healthcare practitioner-AI system, the healthcare practitioner needs to be aware of how the AI system works including its input, model, and output. Historically, decision support systems in clinical decision making have not demonstrated improvements in patient outcomes during randomized control trials [29]. However, the ability for computers to efficiently handle multi-modal data and the predictive power of AI systems has improved significantly. Modern decision support systems can now provide personalized healthcare [30] in various domains [31–33]. AI-enabled support for clinical decision-making based on imaging (e.g., X-ray, mammogram) is particularly advanced. De Fauw et al. [34] propose a referral recommendation whose performance in diagnosing retinal disease reaches or exceeds that of experts on a range of visually impairing retinal diseases. In cardiology, the interpretation of echocardiograms using ML has recently shown considerable potential [35]. ML has also been employed to identify genotypes associated with common symptoms of heart disease [36, 37]. While these support systems have been promising, personalized cardiovascular medicine delivered by AI can go beyond simple image interpretation and genotype association.

10.3.1.2   Exploration

Exploration refers to the use of AI systems to explore new biological processes and aid scientific understanding of medicine [38, 39]. In exploration, healthcare practitioners need to guide AI systems to answer noteworthy questions: Is there a relationship that a practitioner wants to test? Is there a pattern in phenotypic data that one can mine from genomic data? Poplin et al. [40] were able to make hypotheses about risk factors for cardiovascular disease using retinal fundus photographs. The implemented ML model extracted unforeseen features of importance when predicting cardiovascular risk factors: this augments the ability of a healthcare practitioner by directing future research and guiding diagnostic practices.

Exploration aims to verify conjectures that healthcare practitioners have based on experience. The main paradigms of learning for exploration are supervised and reinforcement learning. Exploration takes advantage of the massive amount of patient data recorded in health records and collected during clinical trials. Supervised learning can extract behavioral insights from sensor-collected data, e.g., heart monitors.

Exploration
A study of participant-reported physical activity and sleep duration from a wrist activity monitor was used [41] to train a ML model that identified the activity the participant was engaged in. Ground-truth data was acquired from a camera, which was annotated with the activity of interest providing ground truth labels for supervised learning. The model identifies high-level trends in lifestyle health behaviors, which the authors suggest can influence future public health guidelines.

10.3.1.3 Discovery

In discovery, AI can help reveal unknown patterns and motivate healthcare practitioners to develop randomized control trials to verify patterns observed in the data. Healthcare practitioners can provide guidelines that dictate what data is fed into the AI system and how the discoveries are made. Some relevant questions might be: Is there a space of potential drugs in a large search space (i.e., the space of all possible chemical compounds) wherein one may find a cure? Is there a pattern one can learn from clustering similar data together?

Discovery aims to reveal unknown patterns within large datasets [42]. Differing characteristics across subgroups enable AI systems to model their underlying distinctions. Sometimes the patterns mined from the data could lead to new scientific discoveries.

> **Discovery**
> A genomic score was created [43] to stratify individuals based on their risk trajectories for coronary artery disease. Based on an ML model, they suggested early life genomic screening as an additional risk assessment tool for coronary artery disease. The ability to develop a genomic score, which has practical utility, lies in advances in genome sequencing and lies in AI for genomics. Recent work has also found that AI can be used for discovering novel "genotypes and phenotypes in heterogeneous cardiovascular diseases, such as Brugada syndrome, HFpEF, Takotsubo cardiomyopathy, HTN, pulmonary hypertension, familial atrial fibrillation, and metabolic syndrome" [44].

10.4 Trustworthiness Mechanisms

AI systems can either deliver or fail on the task at hand. In successful cases, people expect AI to act in a verifiably correct and predictable manner; such behavior highlights the trustworthiness of AI. In the case of failure, people should hold an AI accountable for its actions: either AI should transparently provide explanations for why it did what it did, or it should convey its limitations a priori. Trustworthiness ensures systems are predictable, transparent, and robust. It is comprised of competence, reliability, and honesty [45].

Transparency is a mechanism via which AI systems can display their trustworthiness to stakeholders. It allows stakeholders to audit systems to see if the system behaves as desired. Transparency into the training procedures/setup and into AI system innards are equally important.

10.4.1 Predictability

Imagine a diagnostic AI system that leverages electronic health records to make suggested diagnoses to healthcare practitioners [46]. If the system performs well over time (that is, provides the correct diagnosis most of the time) the healthcare practitioners will begin to view the system's behavior as predictably correct and trustworthy. As long as an AI system can convey why it has failed, healthcare practitioners are likely to accept an under-performing AI system [47]. Predictability captures the ability for the AI system to correctly complete the task it was trained to do. Predictable AI systems behave in line with a stakeholder's mental model. Repeat interactions with AI systems help foster trust between the system and the practitioner [48]. The AI system may be uncertain upon seeing a new patient that is unlike any patients in the training set. When faced with this new example, it is important that the system communicates its predictive uncertainty of its diagnosis with the healthcare practitioner [49]. In order to build a trustworthy relationship with healthcare practitioners, AI systems ought to account for real-world uncertainties in deployment. In the face of uncertainty, the healthcare practitioner making a decision can intervene and revert to their clinical judgement.

The AI community has developed algorithms that may be suitable for conveying this predictive uncertainty to non-ML-expert stakeholders [50–53]. If a traditional AI system was tasked with predicting if a chest X-ray had pneumonia or not (two options), these newer systems include a third option, a reject option (also called abstain option or colloquially an "I don't know" option [54]. Selective prediction (also known as reject option classification or learning with abstention) could have large promise in clinical decision making [55]. When an AI system is ambiguous, it is important it defers to healthcare practitioners, who can leverage their expertise to make a decision accordingly.

10.4.2   Procedural Transparency

Procedural transparency entails conveying information about how an AI system is trained [56]. It may expose proprietary information, however disclosures like these can help healthcare practitioners understand the functionalities and limitations of the AI systems in question. Procedural transparency is paramount to building practitioner-AI trust and to ensuring safe adoption of AI in healthcare. Procedural Transparency includes properties of the model used (developers, version, licensing, etc.), intended use cases for the model (primary use, out-of-scope use cases, intended users), details about the training data used (diversity, preprocessing, feature selection), performance metrics (decision thresholds, qualitative results, unitary/intersectional analyses), and ethical considerations [57–60].

10.4.3   Algorithmic Transparency

Algorithmic transparency generally refers to explainability, but also encompasses other concepts such as uncertainty [61]. Algorithmic transparency can provide information on a global level that summarizes the model behavior for multiple data points or the entire training dataset. Algorithmic transparency can also provide information on a local level explaining an individual prediction [62] via multiple methods. Feature importance asks which features are important to the model when doing prediction [63–65]. Sample importance answers which training points were most important to a particular prediction [66–68]. Counterfactual explanations note what needs to change in an input in order to change the outcome [69–71]. Explainability develops models that provide information about how the model came to its decision [72]. One study interviewed healthcare practitioners to explore their clinical decision-making in practice. The participants were given a case study [47] where an ML model was embedded in the electronic health record system and monitored patients in the ICU to assess the likelihood that they would experience cardiac arrest. The practitioners prioritized identifying any discrepancies between the subset of input features responsible for the model's outcome (feature importance) and their clinical judgement.

Explainability can also be applied to augment a healthcare practitioner's decision-making and analysis, such as echocardiogram interpretation. Alsharqi et al. [73] were able to use ML to efficiently, accurately, and reliably interpret echocardiograms, with performance comparable to that of a clinician alone. Zhang et al. [74] were able to support serial patient tracking and analyze echocardiograms on a large scale using a novel analysis pipeline, including identification, image segmentation, structure and function quantification, and disease detection. Their model was able to successfully segment cardiac chambers using a convolutional neural network trained per the segmentation method.

Algorithm

Research in deep learning for medical diagnostics has also developed explanations that reason like clinicians [75]. Similar to how a ML model uses input features to reach an output, medical professionals learn how to proactively search for risk predictors upon seeing a patient [76]. Research in AI is now trying to mirror how medical professionals use current data as well as past experiences with patients to inform decision making. For example, if a doctor treated a rare disease over a decade ago, then that patient can be crucial when attributes alone are uninformative about how a doctor should proceed [77]. This is the equivalent to using "close" training points (past patients) to explain an unseen test point (current patient) [78]. Thus, algorithmic transparency provides much promise in healthcare.

10.4.4   Robustness

In addition to transparency and predictability, AI systems must be robust to shifts in input distributions [79] and to adversarial attacks [80]. Robustness is a system's ability to withstand outliers and other variation during system deployment Distribution shift refers to when the inputs received in deployment differ from the inputs that the AI system was trained on. Covariate shift captures what happens when the input features differ from training to testing [79]. Label shift refers to when the output distributions vary from training to test [79]. For example, if a ML model is trained on geriatric patients but then deployed in the neonatal ward, the model may not perform as expected on younger patients. In some cases, the effects of age may be negligible to the model; however, it is important for the healthcare practitioner to clarify if such a shift is acceptable. While it is possible to create a model for a specific task or problem, recent work has shown that a hospital-specific approach with tailored models for each institution is the most efficient way to robustly augment clinician performance [81]. Since hospitals usually have unique systems for electronic health records, one model may not generalize from one hospital to another.

10.5   Artificial Intelligence Alongside Healthcare Practitioners

Healthcare practitioners play a pivotal role in building and deploying trustworthy AI systems [82]. They can intervene in input engineering, model development, clinical deployment, and model correction.

10.5.1   Input Engineering

Healthcare professionals are essential in ensuring that the inputs and features learned by an AI system are biologically relevant and feasible. They are most familiar with context specific information and can help fill in the gaps where the training data might be lacking. The combination of data analysis and clinical intuition plays a fundamental role in cardiovascular disease management. Input engineering can incorporate human domain expertise into the learning process through collaboration with cardiovascular clinicians.

10.5.2   Model Development

As ML engineers develop models for use in medical contexts, healthcare professionals have the opportunity to assist in model development. Most importantly, healthcare professionals can help with verifying what the model has learnt is biologically relevant by inspecting the explanation generated for its predictions. In healthcare, these techniques can pave the way for clinicians to actively participate in the model selection and to ensure that ultimately the model not only quantitatively be accurate but also it is qualitatively relevant. Feature engineering, where the expertise of the domain experts is considered in what the model pays the most attention to is another way of having healthcare professionals involved in model development [83].

10.5.3 Clinical Deployment

Having clinical experts integrally involved in developing models and engineering the input that feeds the model plays an important role in the trustworthiness of the developed system. Upon AI deployment, healthcare practitioners should use their clinical judgment about the system's recommendation and whether it should be taken, rejected or adjusted. Conveying the degree of predictive certainty by the clinical decision support system when making a prediction can guide this judgment, especially if the system is equipped with explanation facilities. Such explanation techniques facilitate the interaction of the users with the system to gain more insight into the recommendation proposed and to subsequently trust it. Such interactions can help the system self-correct and learn from the adjustment or overrides administered by experts [84].

10.5.4 Model Correction

If a deployed AI system contains errors, there is an opportunity for a healthcare practitioner to intervene and correct the systems' behavior. The learned models may have high accuracy but can accidentally learn spurious correlations between features (that is, the true signal might be masked by noise in the data) [85]. Interactive ML comes to the rescue to involve healthcare practitioners directly in the model correction phase. Enabling healthcare practitioners to identify how to correct the errors (or how to change the model's reasoning on specific inputs) is crucial to successful deployment of AI systems in healthcare.

10.6 Conclusion

The potential of AI in healthcare is limitless. By encouraging interaction between healthcare practitioners and AI systems, society unlocks more potential since AI extends a healthcare practitioner's acumen with the predictive power of machines. Aligned with core human values, an AI system earns a healthcare practitioner's trust and gives them the agency to do more. While current applications of AI systems in clinical settings are limited to ML-driven systems, AI systems can be used to explore more than just datasets for insights. They can be used to discover new drugs or treatments, or to provide decision support to practitioners. For an AI system to show its trustworthiness to healthcare practitioners, the AI system must display predictability, procedural transparency, algorithmic transparency, and robustness. Healthcare practitioners are essential to the successful deployment of AI systems: they can engineer inputs to feed into models, can guide model selection, can assess models in deployment (overriding as needed), and can correct model behavior. The merit of AI in healthcare comes from AI deployed responsibly with the healthcare practitioner in mind.

Acknowledgments   UB acknowledges support from DeepMind and the Leverhulme Trust via the Leverhulme Centre for the Future of Intelligence and from the Partnership on AI.

References

1. Grace K, Salvatier J, Dafoe A, Zhang B, Evans O. When will AI exceed human performance? evidence from AI experts. J Artif Intell Res. 2018;62:729–54.
2. Yu K-H, Beam AL, Kohane IS. Artificial intelligence in healthcare. Nat Biomed Eng. 2018;2(10):719–31.
3. LaRosa E, Danks D. Impacts on trust of healthcare AI. In: Proceedings of the 2018 AAAI/ACM Conference on AI, Ethics, and Society, ACM; 2018. p. 210–5.
4. McCarthy J, Minsky ML, Rochester N, Shannon CE. A proposal for the Dartmouth summer research project on artificial intelligence, August 31, 1955. AI Mag. 2006;27(4):12.
5. Engelbart DC. Augmenting human intellect: a conceptual framework, Menlo Park, CA. 1962.
6. Pasquinelli M. Augmented intelligence. Critical keywords for the digital humanities. 2014.
7. Lucas P, van der Gaag L. Principles of expert systems. Boston (MA): Addison-Wesley Longman Publishing Co., Inc.; 1991.
8. Ledley RS, Lusted LB. Reasoning foundations of medical diagnosis symbolic logic, probability, and value theory aid our understanding of how physicians reason. Science. 1959;130(3366):9–21.
9. Shortlie E, Buchanan B. A model of inexact reasoning in medicine. Math Biosci. 1975;23:351–79.
10. Bishop CM. Pattern recognition and machine learning. New York: Springer; 2006.
11. Rajpurkar P, Irvin J, Zhu K, Yang B, Mehta H, Duan T, Ding D, Bagul A, Langlotz C, Shpanskaya K, et al. Chexnet: radiologist-level pneumonia detection on chest x-rays with deep learning. arXiv [Preprint] arXiv:1711.05225. 2017.
12. Choi D-J, Park JJ, Taqdir A, Lee S. Artificial intelligence for the diagnosis of heart failure. NPJ Digit Med. 2020;3:54.
13. The Gene Ontology Consortium. The gene ontology resource: 20 years and still going strong. Nucleic Acids Res. 2018;47(D1):D330–8.
14. Jaber MI, Song B, Taylor C, et al. A deep learning image-based intrinsic molecular subtype classier of breast tumors reveals tumor heterogeneity that may a detect survival. Breast Cancer Res. 2020;22:12.
15. Ma T, Zhang A. Incorporating biological knowledge with factor graph neural network for interpretable deep learning. arXiv [Preprint] arXiv:1906.00537. 2019. p. 11.
16. Crawford J, Greene CS. Incorporating biological structure into machine learning models in biomedicine. Curr Opin Biotechnol. 2020;63:126–34.
17. Rhee S, Seo S, and Kim S. Hybrid approach of relation network and localized graph convolutional ltering for breast cancer subtype classification. In: Proceedings of the 27th International Joint Conference on Artificial Intelligence, IJCAI'18; AAAI Press; 2018. p. 3527–34
18. Raza K, Singh NK. A tour of unsupervised deep learning for medical image analysis. arXiv [Preprint] arXiv:1812.07715. 2018.

19. Alashwal H, El Halaby M, Crouse JJ, Abdalla A, Moustafa AA. The application of unsupervised clustering methods to alzheimer's disease. Front Comput Neurosci. 2019;13:31.
20. Shah SJ, Katz DH, Deo RC. Phenotypic spectrum of heart failure with preserved ejection fraction. Heart Fail Clin. 2014;10(3):407–18.
21. Hedman ÅK, et al. Identification of novel pheno-groups in heart failure with preserved ejection fraction using machine learning. Heart. 2020;106(5):342–9.
22. Yauney G and Shah P. Reinforcement learning with action-derived rewards for chemotherapy and clinical trial dosing regimen selection. In: Proceedings of the 3rd machine learning for healthcare conference, volume 85 of proceedings of machine learning Research; PMLR; 2018. p. 161–226
23. Sutton RT, Pincock D, Baumgart DC, Sadowski DC, Fedorak RN, Kroeker KI. An overview of clinical decision support systems: benefits, risks, and strategies for success. NPJ Digit Med. 2020;3(1):1–10.
24. Yu C, Liu J, Nemati S. Reinforcement learning in healthcare: a survey. arXiv [Preprint] arXiv:1908.08796. 2019.
25. Kuan R. Adopting AI in health care will be slow and difficult. 2019. https: //hbr.org/2019/10/adopting-ai-in-health-care-will-be-slow-and-difficult
26. Oh J, Wang J, Tang S, Sjoding M, Wiens J. Relaxed parameter sharing: Effectively modeling time-varying relationships in clinical time-series. arXiv [Preprint] arXiv:1906.02898. 2019.
27. Goyal D, Syed Z, and Wiens J. Clinically meaningful comparisons over time: an approach to measuring patient similarity based on subsequence alignment. arXiv [Preprint] arXiv:1803.00744. 2018.
28. Rajkomar A, Oren E, Chen K, Dai AM, Hajaj N, Hardt M, Liu PJ, Liu X, Marcus J, Sun M, et al. Scalable and accurate deep learning with electronic health records. NPJ Digit Med. 2018;1(1):18.
29. Anchala R, Pinto MP, Shrou A, Chowdhury R, Sanderson J, Johnson L, Blanco P, Prabhakaran D, Franco OH. The role of Decision Support System (DSS) in prevention of cardiovascular disease: a systematic review and meta-analysis. PLoS One. 2012;7(10):e47064.
30. Yoon J, Davtyan C, van der Schaar M. Discovery and clinical decision support for personalized healthcare. IEEE J Biomed Health Inform. 2016;21(4):1133–45.
31. Epstein AS, Zauderer MG, Gucalp A, Seidman AD, Caroline A, Fu J, Keesing J, Hsiao F, Megerian M, Eggebraaten T, et al. Next steps for IBM Watson oncology: scalability to additional malignancies. 2014.
32. Gilbert FJ, Astley SM, McGee MA, Gillan MGC, Boggis CRM, Griths PM, Duy SW. Single reading with computer-aided detection and double reading of screening mammograms in the United Kingdom National Breast Screening Program. Radiology. 2006;241(1):47–53.
33. Baek J-H, Ahn S-M, Urman A, Kim YS, Ahn HK, Won PS, Lee W-S, Sym SJ, Park HK, Chun Y-S, et al. Use of a cognitive computing system for treatment of colon and gastric cancer in South Korea. J Clinical Oncol. 2017;35
34. De Fauw J, Ledsam JR, Romera-Paredes B, Nikolov S, Tomasev N, Blackwell S, Askham H, Glorot X, O'Donoghue B, Visentin D, et al. Clinically applicable deep learning for diagnosis and referral in retinal disease. Nat Med. 2018;24(9):1342–50.
35. Ghorbani A, Ouyang D, Abid A, et al. Deep learning interpretation of echocardiograms. NPJ Digit Med. 2020;3:10.
36. Oguz C, Sen SK, Davis AR, Fu Y-P, O'Donnell CJ, Gibbons GH. Genotype-driven identification of a molecular network predictive of advanced coronary calcium in ClinSeq® and Framingham Heart Study cohorts. BMC Syst Biol. 2017;11(1):99.
37. Burghardt TP, Ajtai K. Neural/bayes network predictor for inheritable cardiac disease pathogenicity and phenotype. J Mol Cell Cardiol. 2018;119:19–27.
38. Shickel B, Tighe PJ, Bihorac A, Rashidi P. Deep EHR: a survey of recent advances in deep learning techniques for electronic health record (EHR) analysis. IEEE J Biomed Health Inform. 2017;22(5):1589–604.
39. Gil Y, Greaves M, Hendler J, Hirsh H. Amplify scientific discovery with artificial intelligence. Science. 2014;346(6206):171–2.

40. Poplin R, Varadarajan AV, Blumer K, Liu Y, McConnell MV, Corrado GS, Peng LH, Webster DR. Prediction of cardiovascular risk factors from retinal fundus photographs via deep learning. Nat Biomed Eng. 2018;2:158–64.
41. Willetts M, Hollowell S, Aslett L, Holmes C, Doherty A. Statistical machine learning of sleep and physical activity phenotypes from sensor data in 96,220 UK biobank participants. Sci Rep. 2018;8(1):1–10.
42. Chen H, Engkvist O, Wang Y, Olivecrona M, Blaschke T. The rise of deep learning in drug discovery. Drug Discov Today. 2018;23(6):1241–50.
43. Inouye M, Abraham G, Nelson CP, Wood AM, Sweeting MJ, Dudbridge F, Lai FY, Kaptoge S, Brozynska M, Wang T, Ye S, Webb TR, Rutter MK, Tzoulaki I, Patel RS, Loos RJF, Keavney B, Hemingway H, Thompson J, Watkins H, Deloukas P, Emanuele Di Angelantonio, Adam S. Butterworth, John Danesh, Nilesh J. Samani, and . Genomic risk prediction of coronary artery disease in 480,000 adults. J Am Coll Cardiol, 72(16):1883–1893, 2018. ISSN 0735–1097. doi: https://doi.org/10.1016/j.jacc.2018.07.079. https://www.onlinejacc.org/content/72/16/1883
44. Krittanawong C, Zhang H, Wang Z, Aydar M, Kitai T. Artificial intelligence in precision cardiovascular medicine. J Am Coll Cardiol. 2017;69(21):2657–64.
45. O'Neill O. Linking trust to trustworthiness. Int J Philos Stud. 2018;26(2):293–300.
46. Choi E, Bahadori MT, Schuetz A, Stewart WF, Sun J. Doctor AI: predicting clinical events via recurrent neural networks. In: Machine Learning for Healthcare Conference; 2016. p. 301–18
47. Tonekaboni S, Joshi S, McCradden MD, Goldenberg A. What clinicians want: contextualizing explainable machine learning for clinical end use. In: Machine learning for healthcare conference; 2019. p. 359–80
48. Ferrario A, Loi M, Vigano E. In AI we trust incrementally: a multi-layer model of trust to analyze human-artificial intelligence interactions. Philos Technol. 2019:1–17.
49. Kale A, Kay M, and Hullman J. Decision-making under uncertainty in research synthesis: designing for the garden of forking paths. In: Proceedings of the 2019 CHI conference on human factors in computing systems; 2019. p. 1–14.
50. Gal Y, Ghahramani Z. Dropout as a bayesian approximation: representing model uncertainty in deep learning. In: International conference on machine learning; 2016. p. 1050–1059
51. Subbaswamy A, Saria S. Counterfactual normalization: proactively addressing dataset shift using causal mechanisms. In: 34th Conference on Uncertainty in Artificial Intelligence 2018, UAI; Association For Uncertainty in Artificial Intelligence (AUAI). 2018. p. 947–57.
52. Zhang Y, Vera Liao Q, Bellamy RKE. Effect of confidence and explanation on accuracy and trust calibration in AI-assisted decision making. In: Proceedings of the 2020 conference on fairness, accountability, and transparency, FAT* '20; New York, NY, USA, Portland (OR): Association for Computing Machinery; 2020. p. 295–305. ISBN 9781450369367. doi: https://doi.org/10.1145/3351095.3372852.
53. Antoran J, Bhatt U, Adel T, Weller A, Hernandez-Lobato JM. Getting a CLUE: a method for explaining uncertainty estimates. arXiv [Preprint] arXiv:2006.06848. 2020.
54. Wiener Y, El-Yaniv R. Agnostic selective classification. In: Advances in neural information processing systems; 2011. p. 1665–1673.
55. Hanczar B, Dougherty ER. Classification with reject option in gene expression data. Bioinformatics. 2008;24(17):1889–95.
56. Selbst AD, Boyd D, Friedler SA, Venkatasubramanian S, Vertesi J. Fairness and abstraction in sociotechnical systems. In: Proceedings of the conference on fairness, accountability, and transparency; 2019. p. 59–68
57. Gebru T, Morgenstern J, Vecchione B, Wortman Vaughan J, Wallach H, Daumee H III, Crawford K. Datasheets for datasets. arXiv [Preprint] arXiv:1803.09010. 2018.
58. Deborah Raji I, Yang J. ABOUT ML: annotation and benchmarking on understanding and transparency of machine learning lifecycles. arXiv [Preprint] arXiv:1912.06166. 2019.
59. Arnold M, RKE B, Hind M, Houde S, Mehta S, Mojsilovic A, Nair R, Natesan Ramamurthy K, Olteanu A, Piorkowski D, et al. Factsheets: increasing trust in ai services through supplier's declarations of conformity. IBM J Res Dev. 2019;63(4/5):6–1.

60. Mitchell M, Wu S, Zaldivar A, Barnes P, Vasserman L, Hutchinson B, Spitzer E, Raji ID, Gebru T. Model cards for model reporting. In: Proceedings of the conference on fairness, accountability, and transparency; 2019. p. 220–9

61. Bhatt U, Xiang A, Sharma S, Weller A, Taly A, Jia Y, Ghosh J, Puri R, Moura JMF, Eckersley P. Explainable machine learning in deployment. In: Proceedings of the 2020 conference on fairness, accountability, and transparency; 2020. p. 648–57.

62. Brundage M, Avin S, Wang J, Beleld H, Krueger G, Hadeld G, Khlaaf H, Yang J, Toner H, Fong R, et al. Toward trustworthy AI development: mechanisms for supporting verifiable claims. arXiv [Preprint] arXiv:2004.07213. 2020.

63. Ribeiro MT, Singh S, Guestrin C. "Why should I trust you?" explaining the predictions of any classier. In: Proceedings of the 22nd ACM SIGKDD international conference on knowledge discovery and data mining; 2016. p. 1135–44

64. Lundberg SM, Lee S-I. A unified approach to interpreting model predictions. In: Advances in neural information processing systems; 2017. p. 4765–74

65. Davis B, Bhatt U, Bhardwaj K, Marculescu R, Moura JMF. On network science and mutual information for explaining deep neural networks. In: ICASSP 2020–2020 IEEE International Conference on Acoustics, Speech and Signal Processing (ICASSP); IEEE; 2020. p. 8399–403

66. Koh PW, Liang P. Understanding black-box predictions via influence functions. In: Proceedings of the 34th International Conference on Machine Learning-Volume 70; JMLR.org; 2017. p. 1885–94.

67. Yeh C-K, Kim JK, Yen IEH, Ravikumar PK. Representer point selection for explaining deep neural networks. In: Advances in neural information processing systems; 2018. p. 9291–301.

68. Khanna R, Kim B, Ghosh J, Koyejo S. Interpreting black box predictions using Fisher kernels. In: The 22nd International Conference on Artificial Intelligence and Statistics; 2019. p. 3382–90

69. Wachter S, Mittelstadt B, Russell C. Counterfactual explanations without opening the black box: automated decisions and the GDPR. Harv J Law Technol. 2018;31(2).

70. Dhurandhar A, Chen P-Y, Luss R, Tu C-C, Ting P, Shanmugam K, Das P. Explanations based on the missing: towards contrastive explanations with pertinent negatives. In: Advances in neural information processing systems; 2018. p. 592–603.

71. Ustun B, Spangher A, Liu Y. Actionable recourse in linear classification. In: Proceedings of the conference on fairness, accountability, and transparency; 2019. p. 10-19,

72. Kwon BC, Choi M-J, Taery Kim J, Choi E, Bin Kim Y, Won SK, Sun J, Choo J. RetainVis: visual analytics with interpretable and interactive recurrent neural networks on electronic medical records. IEEE Trans Vis Comput Graph. 2018;25(1):299–309.

73. Alsharqi M, Woodward WJ, Mumith J-A, Markham D, Upton R, Leeson PT. Artificial intelligence and echocardiography. Echo Res Pract. 2018;5:R115–25.

74. Zhang J, Gajjala S, Agrawal P, Tison GH, Hallock LA, Beussink-Nelson L, Lassen MH, Fan E, Aras MA, Jordan CR, Fleischmann KE, Melisko M, Qasim A, Shah SJ, Bajcsy R, Deo RC. Fully automated echocardiogram interpretation in clinical practice. Circulation. 2018;138:1623–35.

75. Bhatt U, Davis B, Moura JMF. Diagnostic model explanations: a medical narrative. In: AAAI Spring Symposium: interpretable AI for well-being; 2019.

76. Evangelista A, Gallego P, Calvo-Iglesias F, Bermejo J, Robledo-Carmona J, Sanchez V, Saura D, Arnold R, Carro A, Maldonado G, et al. Anatomical and clinical predictors of valve dysfunction and aortic dilation in bicuspid aortic valve disease. Heart. 2018;104(7):566–73.

77. Dorr Goold S, Lipkin M Jr. The doctor–patient relationship: challenges, opportunities, and strategies. J Gen Intern Med. 1999;14(Suppl 1):S26.

78. Bhatt U, Weller A, Moura JMF. Evaluating and aggregating feature-based model explanations. arXiv [Preprint] arXiv:2005.00631. 2020.

79. Quiñonero-Candela J, Sugiyama M, Schwaighofer A, Lawrence ND. Dataset shift in machine learning. Cambridge (MA): The MIT Press; 2009.

80. Finlayson SG, Bowers JD, Ito J, Zittrain JL, Beam AL, Kohane IS. Adversarial attacks on medical machine learning. Science. 2019;363(6433):1287–9.

81. Oh J, Makar M, Fusco C, McCaffrey R, Rao K, Ryan EE, Washer L, West LR, Young VB, Guttag J, et al. A generalizable, data-driven approach to predict daily risk of clostridium difficile infection at two large academic health centers. Infect Control Hosp Epidemiol. 2018;39(4):425–33.
82. Ghassemi M, Pushkarna M, Wexler J, Johnson J, and Varghese P. ClinicalVis: supporting clinical task-focused design evaluation. arXiv [Preprint] arXiv:1810.05798, 2018.
83. Roe KD, Jawa V, Zhang X, Chute CG, Epstein JA, Matelsky J, Shpitser I, Overby Taylor C. Feature engineering with clinical expert knowledge: a case study assessment of machine learning model complexity and performance. PloS One, 2020;15(4) e0231300 .
84. Raghu M, Blumer K, Corrado G, Kleinberg J, Obermeyer Z, Mullainathan S. The algorithmic automation problem: prediction, triage, and human effort. arXiv [Preprint] arXiv:1903.12220. 2019.
85. Kelly CJ, Karthikesalingam A, Suleyman M, Corrado G, King D. Key challenges for delivering clinical impact with artificial intelligence. BMC Med. 2019;17(1):195.

Correction to: Digital Health Solutions and Wearable Devices

Jennifer M. Joe, Jaydeo Kinikar, Monique Smith, Michael J. Carr,
Ethan Bechtel, Stephen Randall, and Leah Ammerman

Corrections to: Chapter 2 in A. B. Bhatt (ed.), *Healthcare Information Technology for Cardiovascular Medicine, Health Informatics*, https://doi.org/10.1007/978-3-030-81030-6_2

This book was inadvertently published with a spelling error in the author's name of chapter 2. The correct name is Jaydeo Kinikar, this has been updated with this correction.

The updated version of this chapter can be found at: https://doi.org/10.1007/978-3-030-81030-6_2

Index

Printed in the United States
by Baker & Taylor Publisher Services